THE PROSTATE CANCER ESSENTIALS FOR SURVIVAL SERIES

ADVANCED IMAGING FOR PROSTATE CANCER

MICHAEL J. DATTOLI, MD

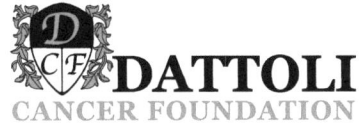

DATTOLI
CANCER FOUNDATION

SARASOTA, FLORIDA

Prostate Cancer Essentials for Survival—Advanced Imaging for Prostate Cancer

Copyright © 2018-2022 by Michael J. Dattoli, M.D.

All rights reserved. No part of this work may be reproduced or transmitted in any form or by any means, electronic or mechanical, including photocopying or recording, or by any information storage or retrieval system, except as may be expressly permitted by the 1976 Copyright Act or in writing by the publisher.

ISBN-13: 978-1-7201-0155-0

Published by the Dattoli Cancer Foundation, Sarasota, FL
Book design and composition by Design Corps, Batavia, IL

MEDICAL DISCLAIMER

This booklet is intended as a supplement but not as a substitute for the medical advice of a physician. It is imperative that you consult a qualified healthcare professional with regard to all matters relating to your health and particular situation. Neither the publisher nor the authors bear responsibility for any consequences due to the reader's decision to use any particular treatment, medication, dietary supplement or other healthcare practices discussed in this book.

DEDICATION

This booklet is dedicated to all those whose lives have been touched by prostate cancer, and to the patients and their families whom we are privileged to serve and educate as cancer care providers.

ACKNOWLEDGMENTS

We are deeply grateful to a number of people who have contributed to this booklet. Our thanks to Greg Lawrence, for his editorial efforts and to Ginya Carnahan, Chris Wells, and Jone Fay at the Dattoli Cancer Center & Brachytherapy Research Institute for their ongoing assistance. We also want to thank Jennifer Cash ARNP, MS, for her long association and many contributions to the Dattoli Cancer Foundation and this booklet series. And we want to thank prostate cancer survivor Bob Hicks for his 3D Color-Flow Power Doppler Ultrasound images.

    We deeply appreciate all of those wonderful patients and family members who have contacted the Dattoli Cancer Foundation for counseling and guidance and in turn have given us their support and encouragement. It is your spirit and commitment in confronting this disease that inspires us all.

CONTENTS

INTRODUCTION

State-of-the-art Imaging for Diagnosis and Treatment 9

OVERVIEW—ADVANCED IMAGING TECHNIQUES

The Advantages of 3D Color-Flow Power Doppler Ultrasound 11
Dattoli Team Biopsy Results with 3D Color-Flow Power Doppler Ultrasound 13
DART, Brachytherapy and 4D IG-IMRT 16
The Art of Interpreting TRUS Images 18
CT Scans and Magnetic Resonance Imaging (MRI) 19
What are Multiparametric MRI and PI-RADS Analysis 22
What is a Bone Scan? 26

APPENDICES

A: Abstracts and References 27
B: Advanced Imaging and Treatment Planning at the Dattoli Cancer Center 43
C: Deciding What is Best for You 51
D: Glossary of Medical Terms 53
E: The Warning Signs of Prostate Cancer 67

About the Author 68
The Dattoli Cancer Foundation Mission 69
Order More Booklets in the Series 70

INTRODUCTION

STATE-OF-THE-ART IMAGING FOR DIAGNOSIS AND TREATMENT

At the Dattoli Cancer Center & Brachytherapy Research Institute, we use the most advanced form of transrectal ultrasound (TRUS), technically referred to as 3-Dimensional Color-Flow Power Doppler Ultrasound (3DCFPDU). This cutting edge innovation has brought a new perspective to diagnosing and treating prostate cancers during recent years. The Doppler technology can reveal areas of brilliant color that are associated with increased blood flow within the gland, identifying sites of suspected tumor growth.

In addition to its use as a diagnostic and monitoring tool, ultrasound plays an essential role in treatments such as brachytherapy (seed implants) and Dynamic Adaptive Radiotherapy (DART) utilizing all modalities associated with 4D Image-Guided Intensity Modulated Radiation Therapy (4D IG-IMRT). With seeding, the needles that are used to insert the seeds are guided by real-time ultrasound images that allow for accurate placement. It is fair to say that the success of prostate brachytherapy over the past two decades has largely been due to the precision of ultrasound-guided needle insertion.

Essentially, 3D Color-Flow Power Doppler Ultrasound is the same kind of technology used to track weather. The term "Doppler" derives from the 19th century physicist Christian Doppler, who determined the perceived wavelength shift relative to velocity between a wave source and observer. For example, we have all experienced the change in pitch of sound from a passing train whistle. 3D Color-Flow Power Doppler Ultrasound images display relative motion of objects in the field of the ultrasound probe which sends and receives the wave pulses.

The visual information obtained by Color-Flow Power Doppler TRUS is profoundly important in planning a prostate biopsy, as it gives the physician color "targets" for the biopsy core samples. Without this advanced imaging, randomly spaced biopsy cores guided by conventional gray-scale ultrasound often miss a cancer entirely, and subject the patient to repeat biopsies as the PSA level continues to rise. Using the older technologies, precious time can be lost as inaccurate, costly and painful biopsies are repeated.

The purpose of this booklet is to help you understand the significance of 3D Color-Flow Power Doppler Ultrasound imaging and how to interpret your results, especially if you are a newly diagnosed patient trying to decide which form of treatment may be right for you. An appreciation of the advantages of 3D Color-Flow Power Doppler Ultrasound, as you consult with your doctor, can help you to make informed decisions that may very well save your life and your quality of life.

In addition, this booklet describes other advanced imaging techniques including magnetic resonance imaging (Dynamic Contrast Enhanced MRI–or DCE-MRI– spectroscopic MRI, endorectal MRI), CT / PET Fusion, Feraheme-USPIO and related techniques that utilize other contrast imaging agents. All of these innovative modalities allow us to improve diagnoses and local staging, determine how extensive and aggressive the cancer is, as well as detecting lymph node metastases and instances of recurrence after primary treatment.

Interpreted wisely in light of a number of related laboratory tests, 3D Color-Flow Power Doppler Ultrasound and various 'fusion' techniques (combining imaging modalities with state-of-the-art computer programs) are powerful tools for making choices about when to treat, when not to treat, and which forms of treatment may be most effective in each individual case. It should be noted that before deciding on any course of treatment, you should fully investigate the likelihood of cure and the risk of side effects that may alter your quality of life. These are the most important considerations in deciding on therapy. Given your age and overall health, you will want to find a balance between treatment effectiveness and side effects–a balance with which you are comfortable, that you can live with both before and after treatment. Knowing what to expect each step of the way is one of the keys to fighting this disease.

As members of the Dattoli Cancer Team, our shared goal with this booklet is to help you make informed decisions. Don't delegate those decisions to someone else. After all, it's your body and your health that are at stake. As you gather information, always consider the source and use your own judgment about your personal needs. *You will know best what is right for you.* Don't be afraid to voice your concerns to your doctor and don't hesitate to ask questions—you have every right to know the answers and to expect a standard of care with which you are satisfied.

–Michael J. Dattoli, M.D.

OVERVIEW

ADVANCED IMAGING TECHNIQUES

The Advantages of 3D Color-Flow Power Doppler Ultrasound

At the Dattoli Cancer Center, we use the most sophisticated 3D Color-Flow Power Doppler Ultrasound scanner with a custom "true" three-dimensional application. Technically referred to as transrectal ultrasonography (TRUS), this is a technique that projects sound waves off the prostate and surrounding organs to create real-time images. The sound waves are generated by a small probe placed inside the rectum. Transrectal ultrasound imaging can in many cases accurately identify the local spread of cancer through the prostate capsule. The technique is also used for real-time guidance in conjunction with seed implants, external radiation therapy, and other treatments.

At our center we have 2 Hitachi 3DCFPD TRUS machines which cost upwards of a million dollars each. We have documented 97% predictive accuracy to diagnose prostate cancer with 3D Color-Flow Power Doppler Ultrasound-guided biopsies.

To make these imaging techniques perfect, we are now fusing multiparametric MRI images (with a 3-Tesla magnet, see below) and 3DCFP TRUS. The outcome of fusing these techniques has been 100% accuracy.

We use 3D Color-Flow Power Dopple Ultrasound and Tissue Harmonic Technology because they provide enhanced visualization and greater definition compared to the conventional gray-scale technique. While there is an art to interpreting 3D Color-Flow Power Doppler images, tumors tend to show increased blood flow or hypervascularity as findings consistent with malignancy. Tumors are growing faster than normal prostate cells and require more blood to support their growth. Tumors therefore tend to create blood vessels around them as they grow, and these can often be identified by 3D Color-Flow Power Doppler Ultrasound.

A conventional TRUS typically shows what are called hypoechogenic areas, which are darker shades of gray. A 3D Color-Flow Power Doppler Ultrasound may show the same image, but provides additional insight into how much perfusion of blood is going into the region, and can reveal whether just one prostate nodule is involved or if there is more cancer dispersed throughout the gland (see images in Appendix B: "Advanced Imaging and Treatment Planning at the Dattoli Cancer Center & Brachytherapy Institute"). It should be noted that the Color-Flow Power Doppler technique is not perfect. There is about a 20-percent false negative rate because some cancer tumors grow so slowly they cannot be detected.

The prostate gland has mostly small capillary vessels, so we normally don't see a lot of color flow on the screen. We know where there should and should not be blood flow in the gland. The larger blood vessels run through the transitional and central zones of the prostate, so we expect to see more blood flow there. Because there is more vascularity through the inner gland, it can be more difficult to detect tumors located there than in the outer gland. The vascularity near the edges of the gland is minimal because there are only micro-vessels in that area.

On a healthy prostate, we shouldn't see color flow near the periphery of the prostate. We are suspicious when we see color flow in that outer region, though it may not necessarily indicate cancer, as the increased vascularity may be the result of inflammation. Only a biopsy tissue sample can confirm the presence of cancer. Following Dynamic Adaptive Radiotherapy (DART) and/or seed implantation, we typically wait at least 6 months before having patients undergo a follow up 3D Color-Flow Power Doppler Ultrasound study, in order to allow any radiation-induced inflammation to be resolved.

Newly developed Tissue Harmonic Technology improves spatial resolution to allow for discrimination of smaller objects and improves contrast resolution to discern very subtle differences in gray-scale images. This is different from conventional TRUS imaging, which generates a pulse of sound and listens for that pulse to echo off structures in the body. With the Tissue Harmonic technology, instead of listening for the same pulse of sound to return in the echo, the ultrasound equipment listens only for a sound pulse at twice the transmitted frequency. The time it takes for the echo to return is proportional to the distance traveled by the sound wave.

A unique 3-D application gives us the ability to rotate these images in the computer, displaying the most accurate and complete picture of the prostate gland and surrounding organs. Our center was the first in the world to adapt this 3-D program to Color-Flow Power Doppler Ultrasound equipment for the diagnosis and treatment of prostate cancer.

As good as the 3D Color-Flow Power Doppler Ultrasound is, until recent years it was not able to give a complete picture of the gland because of its two-dimensional nature and limited 3-D capabilities. With the addition of a new state-of-the-art Sonocubic computer program, we are now able to look at the Doppler images in true 3-D. Areas of suspected tumor growth can be fully assessed from 360 degrees using this pioneering software. A three-dimensional and transparent model of the man's prostate is created by the computer, adding greatly to the information needed prior to performing the all important biopsy. This model can be rotated on the monitor to view the transparent structure from all sides over time—in effect, making the technology 4-D.

Dattoli Team Biopsy Results with 3D Color-Flow Power Doppler Ultrasound

When doing biopsies at our center, in order to guide the biopsy needles to take samples from the prostate, as mentioned, we use both the conventional grayscale ultrasound and 3D Color-Flow Power Doppler Ultrasound (3D-CFPDU). Most patients at other medical centers are biopsied using only the grayscale ultrasound, which is a piece of technology that costs about $40,000, whereas the Color-flow Doppler ultrasound equipment costs many times that. The high cost is one of the reasons 3D Color-Flow Power Doppler Ultrasound is not yet widely available.

With grayscale ultrasound guidance, standard biopsies randomly sample 10 to 12 cores. And we have seen patients with rising PSAs who come to us after having been biopsied elsewhere for several years with negative results. When they come to our center for 3D Color-Flow Power Doppler Ultrasound-guided biopsies, it is not uncommon for us to find 10 to 12 positive cores because the Color-flow Doppler technology is far more discerning than grayscale ultrasound. We have demonstrated that with our own studies.

On February 26th, 2015 in Orlando, Florida, at the annual national Genitourinary Cancers Symposium sponsored by the American Society of Clinical Oncology, we presented a study on prostate biopsies using both grayscale and 3-Dimensional Color-flow Power Doppler Ultrasound (3D-CFPDU). See the full reference (#12) in Appendix A for the content of the presentation.

To summarize our results, we showed that the standard grayscale ultrasound biopsies often lead to sampling errors with mixed diagnosis, delayed diagnosis and the need for repeated biopsies, under-staging, and finding indolent (very slow growing) prostate cancers that often leads to over-treatment. We also pointed out in our study that infections are common with the standard biopsy. The standard approach is to perform the biopsy through the rectal wall, and that approach carries the risk of introducing rectal flora into the bloodstream. That can lead to sepsis, which is a systemic infection, and many patients end up requiring hospitalization when that occurs.

But we reduce the risk of infection and avoid that by using a sterile, transperineal approach to biopsies that is similar to the way we perform brachytherapy seed implants. And our patients are under anesthesia for this procedure. Instead of entering through the rectum with needles, we enter through the perineum, which is the area between the scrotum and anus. We also extend the patient's legs to the dorso-lithotomy position, which gives us much greater access to the prostate. With the standard biopsy, the patient is on his side and the physician is limited by having to go through the rectum with a biopsy gun and is thus unable to sample the entire gland. This is especially limiting with patients who have large glands. With the extended dorso-lithotomy position that we use, the patient is supine with the pelvic arch open so we can more easily take our needle samples directly from the prostate, and we have access to the entire gland even with patients who have enlarged glands due to BPH.

One other advantage of using the transperineal approach is that we know exactly where each core sample comes from, because each needle enters through a template that precisely allows us to map the position. Once we have the pathology results, we will know exactly where the cancer is located and can carry out treatments as needed with brachytherapy and DART with great accuracy.

As you will see, our study followed 192 patients, and we divided them into four groups. All but two of the patients had been biopsied previously using grayscale ultrasound. The first group of patients was termed hypoechoic, meaning the visible lesion was seen as a dark area in the ultrasound image. A second group was hypervascular, meaning the lesion was colorful in the image. A third group was hypoechoic with hypervascular pulsatile vessels, meaning the lesion was dark but there was a heart rhythm associated with the blood flow that we could see in the image. And a fourth group was characterized as hypoechoic with non-pulsatile vessels, meaning a dark lesion that is not in sync with the patient's heart. That is because those lesions are growing independently.

In the image for the first group, the dark area of the lesion is indicated by arrows. The area might be cancer, but it could be an adenoma or atrophy. The image for the second group shows bright, colorful areas on the right side. The third image shows a dark lesion on the left with a heart rhythm indicated on the right like you might see on an EKG. The fourth group is illustrated by two images, and there is a dark lesion on the left, but no visible heart rhythm – it's flat-lined on the right. There is no visible heart rhythm because the cancer is independent of normal blood flow.

The results reported show that for Groups 1 and 2, the biopsy indicated cancer in about 20% of patients, while Group 3 showed 55% positive biopsy results. But Group 4 came back with 97% positive results, with Glesaon scores 7 to 10.

We concluded that transperineal template-guided biopsies using combined grayscale and 3D Color-Flow Power Doppler Ultrasound are highly effective and also cost-effective in a high volume setting by reducing the number of biopsies and enhancing the detection of serious prostate cancers.

In February 2018, the Dattoli team offered additional research results at the American Society of Clinical Oncology Genitourinary (ASCO GU) Cancers Symposium. The presentation was entitled, "Efficacy of Ferumoxytol (Feraheme) as a Lymphatic Contrast Agent in Prostate Cancer" (see full reference (#1) in Appendix A).

A recent study from the University of Pennsylvania confirmed our published findings and reported that ongoing clinical trials utilizing Feraheme as an MRI contract agent are promising (Repurposing Ferumoxytol: Diagnostic and therapeutic applications of an FDA-approved nanoparticle, Theranostics 2022; 12(2):796-816). These researchers observed, "Moreover, ferumoxytol holds great promise for many other biomedical applications including MRI, drug delivery, oral biofilm treatment, and anti-cancer and anti-inflammatory therapies."

These state-of-the-art imaging techniques can identify lymph node spread in patients initially treated for high-risk disease, and they are already allowing us to effectively treat patients with positive lymph nodes by utilizing DART. Our expectation is to further increase our cure rate in this group of patients by treating lymph nodes which may otherwise have not been detected and located with specificity without the benefit of the USPIO/MRI scanning and/or contrast-enhanced MRI and CT imaging.

These diagnostic advances have tremendous potential for improving overall survival of recurrent prostate cancer patients, and also for identifying and treating otherwise undetected cancer in pelvic and abdominal lymph nodes of patients presenting at first diagnosis with high-risk, aggressive prostate cancer. Such breakthroughs are helping us to determine which cancers are tigers and which are pussycats—which are highly aggressive and which are more contained and more easily treated.

What we are finding is that we can control lymph node disease better with this approach to treatment. In many ways, control can be as effective as cure.

We don't cure diabetes or hypertension or a host of other diseases, but we can control them. So if we can control prostate cancer with these patients who have regionally-advanced disease, we believe they will benefit both in terms of survival and quality of life.

Research studies that have reported our findings to date with USPIO include the following:

> Yun Rose Li, Michael J. Dattoli, Jelle Barentsz, Mack Roach III, *Radiotherapy guided by ultra small superparamagnetic iron oxide (USPIO)-contrast MRI staging for patients with advanced or recurrent prostate cancer*, submitted to the American Society of Clinical Oncology (ASCO) for featured conference presentations in February, 2020 (see Appendix B of this booklet).

> Dattoli MJ, Bravo SM, Kaplon DM, Hayes M, Osorio A, Dycus PM, Bostwick D, Kaminski JM, *Efficacy of Feraheme as Lymphatic Contrast Agent in Prostate Cancer;* featured presentations at the February 2018 annual symposiums of the American Society of Clinical Oncology (ASCO) and the Annual Symposium on Clinical Interventional Oncology (CIO) (see Appendix B of this booklet).

> Bravo, S.M., Dattoli, M.J., Myers, C.E., et al; *Safety and Efficacy of Feraheme as a Lympatic Contrast Agent.* ASTRO Symposia. Atlanta, GA, October 2013.

> Bravo, S.M., Dattoli, M.J., Myers, C.E., et al; *Ferumoxytol as a Lymph Node Contrast Agent in Patients with Metastatic Prostate Carcinoma: Rad-Path Correlation, including presentation.* ASTRO Symposia. Orlando, FL, February 2013.

> Bravo, S.M., Dattoli, M.J. Myers, C.E., et al: *Ferumoxytol as a Lymph Node Contrast Agent in Patients with Metastatic Prostate Carcinoma: Rad-Path Correlation, including presentation,* Radiologic Sciences of North America, Chicago, Illinois, Novermber 2012

> Bravo, S.M., Dattoli, M.J., Myers, C.E., et al; *Potential for Feraheme as Lymphatic Contrast Imagine Agent.* Submitted to RSNA November 2011.

> Bravo, S.M., Dattoli, M.J., Myers, C.E., et al; *Safety of Ferumoxytol (Feraheme) in Patients with Prostate Carcinoma.* Submitted to RSNA November 2011.

> Bravo, S.M., Dattoli, M.J., Myers, C.E., et al; *Ferumoxytol as Lymph Node Contrast Agent in Patients with Metastic Prostate Carcinoma: Rad-Path Correlation.* Submitted to RSNA November 2011.

DART, Brachytherapy and 4D IG-IMRT

For more than four decades, the evolution of radiation delivery technologies has been based upon a single objective: maximize the dose to the tumor while minimizing the dose to surrounding normal tissue (thereby minimizing side effects).

Today the most advanced beam technology available is known as high resolution 4-Dimensional Image-Guided Intensity Modulated Radiation Therapy (4D IG-IMRT). The Dattoli Cancer Center was the first private facility in America to offer it to patients. Using 4D IG-IMRT, we are able to realize the full potential of what is known as "Dynamic Adaptive Radiotherapy" (DART).

DART is a coordinated systems approach made possible by the technological convergence of image-guided tools, which integrate both image and data management while utilizing sophisticated treatment planning capabilities such as "autosegmentation" and "deformable registration"–all for the purpose of optimized IMRT treatment delivery. Such a cutting edge system ties together every step, from 4D IG-IMRT simulation and treatment planning to adaptive treatment delivery based on the reality of a patient's exact treatment "condition" and position each and every day, AS IT CHANGES. It is becoming increasingly well known that changes such as tumor position, size and shape do occur not only during a several week treatment regime, but also on a daily basis.

DART achieves the single most important goal ever achieved in Radiation Treatment: Delivering the exact dose to the exact place at exactly the precise time, every time, even when the target moves, shrinks or changes shape—an extraordinary accomplishment!

The actual implementation of DART relies on handling large volumes of continuously changing patient data, interpreting those changes and then immediately acting upon them in real-time. For example, rather than using a one-size-fits-all approach, physicians are empowered to choose a dose schema (e.g. "boost") at a chosen moment in time and make necessary changes to a treatment plan "on the fly" based on cone-beam image capture that reveals real-time changes in the target as it responds to treatment. The bottom line involves managing the motion and biological changes of the target (tumor) and dynamically adapting the 4D IG-IMRT treatment. This makes for truly "individualized" treatment delivery, which is made possible through advanced imaging technologies.

Although each individual is unique, most patients being treated at our institution receive a treatment protocol of combination therapy, utilizing DART, 4-D IG-IMRT and seed implantation (brachytherapy). These state-of-the art treatment modalities rely on advanced imaging techniques and sophisticated computer software programs.

The resurgence of interest in prostate brachytherapy over the past two decades was primarily driven by the technological innovation of transrectal ultrasound (TRUS), which allows for real time imaging during treatment planning and is also used for monitoring intraoperative needle placement. TRUS imaging is supplemented by computerized tomography (CT) and Dynamic Contrast

Enhanced Magnetic Resonance Imaging (DCE-MRI). Each of the various imaging modalities has its advantages and disadvantages.

TRUS, MRI and CT images all reveal pre-treatment prostate contours and can be used in tandem to determine the number and placement of implant seeds (ie. Palladium-103, Iodine-125). While the appearance of the prostatic and periprostatic regions varies qualitatively between the imaging modalities, the size and shape of the prostate are fairly consistent between techniques when interpreted correctly.

The visualization of prostate margins with these complementary modalities ultimately determines the radioactivity required and where it is placed. The same holds true for DART-modulated IG-IMRT, which is often combined with brachytherapy as the protocol of choice for intermediate and higher risk patients. At our institution, we employ Varian IG-IMRT technology with SonArray Ultrasound-Guided Positioning, online portal imagery, "cone beam" tomography, "Portal Vision," and real-time 4D physician review. These advanced imaging technologies allow for the checks and balances necessary to deliver DART.

The Art of Interpreting TRUS Images

As noted above, we utilize Color-Flow Power Doppler Ultrasound since it provides enhanced visualization and greater definition compared to the conventional grayscale technique (Smeenge et al, Current Open Urol, May 2012, Pinto et al, Urol Int, March 2011, Aigner et al, J. Endourol, May 2010). While there is an art to interpreting 3D Color-Flow Power Doppler images, tumors tend to demonstrate increased perfusion or hypervascularity as findings consistent with malignancy. We have been utilizing Color-Flow Power Doppler technology for the past two decades.

The standard grayscale TRUS shows hypoechogenic areas typically as darker shades of gray. A 3D Color-flow Power Doppler Ultrasound may show the same image, but it provides additional insight into how much perfusion of blood is going into the region and can reveal whether just one prostate nodule is involved or if there is more cancer dispersed throughout the gland.

In addition, biopsies guided by Color-Flow Power Doppler Ultrasound have the advantage of showing the optimal sites from which to secure tissue samples. Many patients who come to our institution have already had biopsies performed elsewhere. Once the initial diagnosis has been established, we typically request that the specimen slides be reviewed again by a pathologist who specializes in prostate pathology.

It should also be noted that prostate volume and shape can change when patients are anesthetized. Volumetric inconsistencies can also stem from physiologic changes. Measured by TRUS or MRI, prostate volume can change from day to day by approximately 10%. This variation is consistent with both modalities and may reflect actual changes in volume rather than inconsistent technique.

The impact of such reproducibility variables on clinical results is unknown. It is possible that miscalculated low volumes could lead to inadequate dose coverage of the prostatic periphery, and miscalculated high volumes could lead to complications due to over-radiation of normal tissue. Such potential problems in treatment planning and evaluation can be effectively avoided by registration and cross-referencing the TRUS, MR and CT imaging techniques. Even with the wide variation in how the modalities are implemented, clinical results with transperineal brachytherapy and DART appear highly favorable. Effective planning and operator skill appear to be the most significant factors of practical consequence.

CT Scans and Magnetic Resonance Imaging (MRI)

The main advantages of the CT scan over the other modalities are that CT offers a finer delineation of sources and more accurate imaging of the pubic bones. In addition, the CT requires less patient preparation and is less operator-dependent than TRUS. The CT scan is widely used for post-implant dosimetry and quality control. The primary disadvantage of CT-based seed implants is the lack of real time imaging. While CT scans provide less defined images of the outer prostatic contour and internal architecture, CT images do accurately delineate the spatial relationship between the prostate, rectum and pubic bones.

More contemporary spiral or helical CT scans provide greater resolution while taking less time to acquire the information. At our institution, a GE High Speed Helical CT Scanner captures high resolution, 3-dimensional images of the prostate, seminal vesicles, bladder, urethra and rectum, which are required to accurately design individual treatment plans. This scanner is also equipped to perform QCT Bone Density evaluations for patients undergoing hormone therapy as part of their treatment protocol.

A University of Washington study compared TRUS and CT volumes drawn independently by three observers (Badiozamani, Wallner and Blasko). They reported the imaging modalities were consistent in measuring anterior-posterior, lateral and cranial-caudal dimensions (Badiozamani et al, Comparability of CT-based and TRUS-based prostate volumes. Int J Radiat Oncol Biol Phys. 1999 Jan 15;43 (2):375-8). The significance of this finding is that CT and TRUS images are actually in close correspondence in determining pre-treatment volumes. When interpreted correctly, the CT and TRUS volumes are interchangeable.

Magnetic Resonance Spectroscopic Imaging (MRSI) is a highly discriminating test in terms of both the internal architecture of the prostate gland and determining whether or not there is extra-prostatic extension. With its high degree of detail, the endorectal MRI can show whether or not there is rectal or seminal vesicle involvement. Bladder invasion can also be detected by an endorectal MRI, while it's not commonly seen with a CT scan or an ultrasound study.

Zaider and colleagues at Memorial Sloan-Kettering reported a biologic-based optimization technique that registers MRI images to intraoperative ultrasound images in order to achieve dose escalation to intraprostatic tumor deposits (Zaider et al, Treatment planning for prostate implants using magnetic-resonance spectroscopy imaging. Int J Radiat Oncol Biol Phys. 2000 Jul 1;47 (4):1085-96). Similarly, Mizowaki and colleagues reported on integrating functional imaging modalities with the registration of MRI to TRUS and CT images (Mizowaki, et al, Towards integrating functional imaging in the treatment of prostate cancer with radiation: the registration of the MR spectroscopy imaging to ultrasound/CT images and its implementation in treatment planning. Int J Radiat Oncol Biol Phys. 2002 Dec 1;54 (5):1558-64).

The endorectal MRI is much like an ultrasound probe in that it is placed in the rectum and allows you to image the prostate very closely. It's as detailed a test as you can get in terms of looking at the capsule of the prostate and determining whether or not there is cancer that has extended outside of the prostate gland. The Dynamic Contrast Enhanced MRI is proving to be superior to the spectroscopic MRI as the true gold standard among the imaging modalities known as Multiparametric MRI. True Multiparametric MRI can have an accuracy rate for detection of more than 90% when it has 3 of the following 5 components: an endo-rectal probe, a 3 Tesla magnet, spectroscopy, dynamic contrast enhancement and what is known as diffusion weighting of the images (see "What are Multiparametric MRI and PI-RADS Analysis?").

At our center, most patients undergo an endorectal MRI (preferably Dynamic Contrast Enhanced MRI) in addition to Color-Flow Power Doppler TRUS and 2.0 mm fine section helical CT prior to prostate brachytherapy and/or DART. The only reason a patient wouldn't have an MRI is if his insurance company doesn't cover it and the patient can't afford the test, as it is expensive. The cost of a diagnostic pelvic MRI can be two to three times higher than the cost for a TRUS or CT. Setting aside cost considerations, the art of advanced radiation planning and design depends in large part on optimal integration of these complementary imaging modalities.

Dynamic Contrast Enhanced MRI calculates both increased vessel permeability and increased cellular density (also called extra-cellular volume), which are key physiological indicators of PCa. 75% accuracy has been reported with DCE-MRI (Bloch, et al, Radiotherapy Oncology, 2003, 66(2): 173-179). This is a very accurate test compared to pathological specimens taken during prostatectomy. As noted above, 3D Color-flow Power Doppler Ultrasound reveals suspicious red areas due to vascularity (blood flow). Normal tissues pulse with blood flow, but cancers don't; they're stagnant, not in sync with the normal circulating blood flow. Dynamic Contrast Enhanced MRI is somewhat similar to 3D Color-Flow Power Doppler Ultrasound. The two tests complement each other.

The use of encapsulated iron oxide nanoparticles or ultrasmall superparamagnetic iron oxide (USPIO) as MRI contrast agents is proving to be quite effective in identifying prostate cancer metastasis in the lymph nodes. Feraheme (Ferumoxytol) is a ferromagnetic nanoparticle which is a modified version of these USPIO MRI contrast agents that shows great promise. When extensive lymph node involvement is detected, we have to use an arsenal of sophisticated techniques that define Dynamic Adaptive Radiotherapy, which allows us to follow the movement of organs and adjust for that natural motion. This allows us to zero in on the target while avoiding surrounding healthy tissue. This degree of accuracy is especially important when treating the pelvic lymph nodes. For a full discussion of USPIO imaging and lymph node disease, please see our Essentials booklet, *Lymph Node Positive Prostate Cancer: Advanced Diagnostics and Treatment*.

Additional staging studies may include ProstaScint® with CT or MRI Fusion. The ProstaScint® Scan is a staging test that utilizes a radioactive isotope attached to a monoclonal antibody (mAb). The isotope targets a specific cancer protein known as prostate specific membrane antigen (PSMA). After this combined isotope-mAb is injected into the bloodstream, it will track down that particular cancer protein and then attach to it. This is an imaging test rather than a blood test, per se. Three to four days after being injected, a patient is scanned with a special camera that picks up the radiation emitted by the isotope and locates the cancer. In view of its high rate of false positives and false negatives, this test is not our first choice in working with patients. Other tests are available at this point that utilize different contrast agents and offer greater predictive accuracy.

Functional multi-modality magnetic resonance imaging includes high resolution MR imaging, Dynamic Contrast Enhanced MRI, MR-spectroscopy (MRS), and diffusion weighted MR imaging (DWI). With functional multi-modality MR imaging, it is possible to detect and exactly locate the tumor (tumors) in the prostate gland with a high degree of accuracy. Taken together, all of these tests enable us to visualize various physical aspects of the prostate, such as its size, shape and contour.

As mentioned, the tests provide us with detailed information about the volume and location of the tumor sites. With this information, we are able to determine the optimal protocol for treating the disease, deriving in advance a unique treatment blueprint for each individual patient. It should be noted that fusion studies are relatively new and are only as good as the technologist performing them and the radiologist interpreting them. Like everything else in this field, it pays to search out experienced practitioners who deal with a large case load of patients.

What are Multiparametric MRI and PI-RADS Analysis?

Multiparametric MRI involves a sequence of imaging techniques that provide detailed anatomical and functional information that is not possible with grey scale ultrasound. Radiologists can use multiparametric MRI to identify the location of a tumor or tumors, to measure the extent of a tumor, and to determine whether a tumor has spread beyond the prostate gland. Multiparametric MRI scanning usually consists of three distinct imaging techniques (parameters): T2-weighted MRI, diffusion-weighted MRI, and Dynamic Contrast Enhanced MRI (DCE-MRI).

A T2-weighted MRI exam provides doctors with anatomic information about the prostate gland. This technique is useful for the detection, localization and staging of prostate cancers. It offers detailed visualizations of the prostate and its three distinct zones:

- The peripheral zone (PZ) contains the most prostatic tissue. The largest area of the peripheral zone is at the back of the gland near the rectal wall. When a doctor performs a digital rectal exam, it is the back of the gland that he is feeling. Approximately 70-80% of prostate cancers originate in the peripheral zone.

- The central zone (CZ) surrounds the ejaculatory ducts. Less than 5% of prostate cancers originate in this zone, and they are often more aggressive and more likely to invade the seminal vesicles.

- The transition zone (TZ) surrounds the urethra where it enters the gland. This area grows in men over the years and is responsible for benign prostatic hyperplasia (BPH). About 20% of prostate cancers originate in this zone.

On T2-weighted MRI images, tumors in the peripheral zone of the prostate typically appear as bright spots against a dark background. Cancers in the transition zone are more difficult to detect. They may appear as smudged charcoal against a dark background. T2-weighted MRI scans are also used to evaluate the seminal vesicles and bladder wall to determine if a tumor has spread beyond the prostate.

Diffusion-weighted imaging (DWI) measures the motion of water molecules within the prostate, which provides useful functional information about cancers. This sequence produces an ADC value for different areas of the prostate gland. ADC values measure the degree of motion through different tissues. Lower ADC values more often in cancerous tissue than in healthy tissue. The ADC values also tend to correlate with Gleason scores, with lower ADC values indicating a higher Gleason score

At our center, approximately 90% of our patients undergo an MRI prior to treatment, preferably Dynamic Contrast Enhanced MRI–or DCE-MRI–which is superior to any other type of MRI currently available (including the spectroscopic MRI–or MRSI). DCE-MRI provides more detailed imaging than MRSI. With the Dynamic Contrast Enhanced MRI, a contrast agent is administered to the patient and is used to evaluate blood flow through the prostate. Cancerous tissue absorbs the contrast agent more quickly than healthy tissue, which is revealed on DCE images. MRI contrast agents such as Feraheme and Combidex are also being utilized to identify lymph node and bone metastases, though their availability in the U.S. is limited (for more on this subject, see the Dattoli Cancer Foundation booklet, *Lymph Node Positive Prostate Cancer: Advanced Diagnostics and Treatment*).

Contrast Enhanced MRI is in some ways similar to Color-Flow Power Doppler Ultrasound. To some extent, the two tests complement each other. When cancer is revealed on the DCE-MRI, we will also see it on ultrasound. However, we also sometimes see tumors on Color-Flow Power Doppler Ultrasound that are missed by MRI scans. Because of the limited view of the prostate gland provided by both MRI and ultrasound imaging, some cancers may be missed on larger glands, those greater than 50 cc. The only reason a patient would not have an MRI in our practice is if his insurance company would not pay for it and the patient can't afford the test, as it is expensive. The cost of a diagnostic pelvic MRI is at least two to three times higher than the cost for a TRUS or CT scan.

Multiparametric MRI studies are interpreted according to the Prostate Imaging Reporting and Data System (PI-RADS, Version 2). This is a classification system that uses a 5-point scale to standardize the evaluation of multiparametric MRI. A PI-RADS interpretation indicates the likelihood of indolent prostate cancer versus clinically significant prostate cancer (intermediate and high-risk cancers) based on the three multiparametric MRI techniques.

PI-RADS 1–Highly unlikely that clinically significant cancer is present.

PI-RADS 2–Unlikely that clinically significant cancer is present.

PI-RADS 3–Uncertain whether clinically significant cancer is present.

PI-RADS 4–Likely that clinically significant cancer is present.

PI-RADS 5–Highly likely that clinically significant cancer is present.

With PI-RADS 4 or 5 results, patients should be recommended for biopsy. For results of PI-RADS 1 or 2, a recommendation for biopsy would likely be inappropriate, though other factors may also be considered. For results of PI-RADS 3, biopsy may be deemed appropriate taking into account a patient's history and preferences in consultation with his physician.

One of the benefits of multiparametric MRI is its ability to help men decide on active surveillance as a management strategy rather than undergoing primary therapies such as radical prostatectomy or radiation therapy. Monitoring men in active surveillance was previously accomplished using only evaluations based on PSA testing and blind biopsy. With multiparametric MRI, doctors are able to better determine which patients are likely to have low-risk, indolent disease rather than intermediate and high-risk disease. This approach allows men with low-risk disease to delay primary therapy and side effects, until there is evidence of disease progression (a rising PSA).

Another important benefit of multiparametric MRI is that it allows for targeted biopsies. Biopsy needles can be guided using real-time MRI images or multiparametric MRI images can be fused with real-time ultrasound images to guide biopsy needles. These procedures are referred to as MRI-guided biopsy and MRI-TRUS fusion biopsy respectively. When PI-RADS evaluation is used to triage men for biopsy, both MRI-guided and MRI-TRUS fusion biopsy offer improved diagnostic outcomes with fewer needles compared to the conventional grey-scale ultrasound-guided biopsy.

A PSA screening program that incorporates multiparametric MRI is likely to improve screening for prostate cancer in a number of ways:

- By reducing the total number of biopsies and total number of biopsy needles used, reducing complications associated with biopsy.
- By improving the diagnostic accuracy of for intermediate and high-risk prostate cancers.
- By reducing the detection of low-risk, indolent prostate cancers.
- By more accurately recommending active surveillance for low-risk patients when appropriate rather than primary treatment.

Once prostate cancer is confirmed by biopsy, that detailed anatomic and functional information provided by multiparametric MRI can help to guide treatment decisions. For instance, multiparametric MRI can effectively identify seminal vesicle invasion, extraprostatic extension and pelvic lymph node involvement.

Patients considering multiparametric MRI are advised to take into account the technology used by different radiology facilities and the experience (or lack of experience) of radiologists interpreting scans. Many studies suggest that multiparametric MRI is more effectively performed with 3T MRI machines. In addition, studies suggest that multiparametric MRI exams are more accurately interpreted by radiologists with extensive experience evaluating these advanced imaging techniques.

A 2014 multinational study compared conventional gray-scale ultrasound-guided biopsies with multiparametric MRI-targeted biopsies with PI-RADS interpretation. Researchers reported the following improved results with multiparametric MRI with PI-RADS:

51% reduction in number of biopsies compared with TRUS.

84% reduction in number of biopsy needles used.

89.4% reduction in detection of low-risk, indolent cancer.

17.7% increase in detection of intermediate- and high-risk cancer.

By using multiparametric MRI and PI-RADS interpretation to selectively guide biopsies in men with elevated PSA, instead of conventional ultrasound-guided biopsy, this study showed a reduction in the need for biopsy while improving overall detection of clinically significant intermediate and high-risk cancers (Pokorny MR, et al, Eur Urol. 2014 Jul;66(1):22-9).

A 2015 study published by researchers at the National Cancer Institute showed even greater improvement with MRI-TRUS fusion-guided biopsies. These researchers reported a reduction of 17% in the detection of low-risk cancers with an increase of 30% in the detection of high risk cancers compared to conventional TRUS-guided biopsies. This study demonstrated that MRI-TRUS fusion biopsy was associated with an increase in the detection of intermediate and high-risk prostate cancers and decreased detection of low-risk, indolent prostate cancers (Okoro C, et al, <u>J Endourol</u>. 2015 Oct;29(10):1115-21).

In addition to reducing the number of biopsies, image-guided biopsies that utilize both the Color-Flow Power Doppler Ultrasound and multiparametric MRI techniques can save lives by improving the efficacy of PSA screening. The bottom line is that doctors utilizing these imaging modalities are better able to determine which patients are not at risk for clinically significant prostate cancer and do not need to undergo biopsies. Some of these low-risk patients may elect to pursue Active Surveillance rather than undergo an aggressive primary treatment such a surgery or radiation.

What is a Bone Scan?

A bone scan is an imaging technique used to detect bone metastases, which appear as "hot spots" on film. It is far more sensitive than conventional x-rays. The bone scan procedure is performed by injecting a small amount of radioactive dye called technetium into the patient's bloodstream. A special camera is then used to photograph the skeleton, and any irritation of the bone will show up as a spot on the image.

If a patient's PSA is high, greater than 10, or if the Gleason score is greater than or equal to 7, then I usually recommend a bone scan. Similarly, a bone scan is also recommended if a patient has a low PSA yet palpable disease and/or a Gleason score suggesting aggressive disease. A spot on a bone scan may be caused by cancer that has metastasized, or by arthritis and other causes. When an abnormality shows up on a bone scan, further tests such as traditional x-rays, CT or MRI may be used to determine if the cause is cancer. It is important to establish a baseline to differentiate between cancer and other abnormalities.

Most of our patients undergo an 18F-FDG Fluoride PET/CT Fusion study, which has a predictive accuracy of 98% (Einat E et al., J Nucl Med 2006; 47:287-297). This avoids the false positive and false negative rates which may be associated with bone scans (as a result of the 18F tumor-imaging agent). Meanwhile, the FDG portion of this test may pick up Gleason 8 to 10 prostate cancers in the lymph nodes, as well as other cancers which may as yet not have been detected in the body (e.g. lung cancers, gastrointestinal malignancies, head and neck cancers, and lymphomas). In addition, 11C-Choline PET/CT is a test currently being used to advantage at the Mayo Clinic.

APPENDIX A

ABSTRACTS AND REFERENCES

1) Dattoli Lymph Node Imaging study. The following abstract was presented at two medical conferences in February 2018, the Annual Symposium on Clinical Interventional Oncology (CIO) and the Genitourinary Cancers Symposium cosponsored by the American Society of Clinical Oncology (ASCO), the American Society for Radiation Oncology (ASTRO), and the Society of Urologic Oncology (SUO).

Efficacy of Feraheme as Lymphatic Contrast Agent in Prostate Cancer

Dattoli MJ, Bravo SM, Kaplon DM, Hayes M, Osorio A, Dycus PM, Bostwick D, Kaminski JM

BACKGROUND: Ferumoxytol (Feraheme), a ferromagnetic nanoparticle with lymphotrophic biokinetics, is delivered to lymph nodes via normal macrophages. MRI suppresses normal lymph nodes containing Feraheme. Objective is to validate the agent's safety and efficacy in finding lymph node positivity in prostate cancer (PCa).

METHODS: Nonrandomized prospective evaluation of 178 consecutive PCa patients (pts) at high risk for prostate lymph node spread were enrolled 2/13-3/15. All received IV Feraheme. 177 received infusion of 6/mg/kg given over 20 minutes. One pt received 3 mg/kg infusion. T2 MEDIC and T2* sequence imaging of the abdomen and pelvis, performed 24 hours later. Images were reviewed by 2 board certified radiologists with same interpretations, blinded to clinical and histo-path information (pre-MRI TNM stage, PSA or Gleason score). Lymph nodes were deemed abnormal if they did not suppress after Feraheme infusion (group 1, 94 patients). Lymph nodes were deemed suspicious by MRI if suppressed and met usual size criteria with high signal intensity on DWI and decreased ADC map values and morphologic features (group 2, 84 pts). 83 group 1 pts had CT biopsies (77 pelvis, 6 retroperitoneum); 11 pts had open PLND. 382 lymph nodes were sampled. 76 group 2 patients had CT biopsies (73 pelvis, 3 retroperitoneum); 9 pts had open PLND. 340 lymph nodes were sampled. Rad-path correlation was performed. Resected nodes were stained; reviewed by a single pathologist with no knowledge of MRI findings. The histo-path results for each node were cataloged for later MRI comparison.

RESULTS: 90 group 1 pts (96%) proved metastatic PCa; 4 pts (4%) were normal. 68 group 1 pts (77%) contained malignant lymph nodes not meeting usual imaging criteria for malignancy. 39 group 2 pts showed metastatic PCa; 46 pts (53%) were normal. One group 2 pt experienced an allergic reaction with hives; infusion ceased at 3mg/kg; pt treated to full resolution with 50 mg IV Benadryl.

CONCLUSION: Feraheme can be used to evaluate for lymphatic dissemination of metastatic disease in PCa patients, with a lower limit of resolution of focal lymph node metastases of 2-3 mm. Improved resolution brings implications for therapeutic radiation planning in setting of newly diagnosed or recurrent/metastatic PCa. Toxicity was very acceptable at 6mg/kg. Feraheme may play a significant role as a lymphatic contrast agent in the early dissemination of lymphatic metastatic disease.

2) Purohit RS, Shinohara K, Meng MV, Carroll PR, Imaging clinically localized prostate cancer. Urol Clin North Am. 2003 May;30(2):279-93.

Department of Urology, 400 Parnassus Avenue, A632, University of California-San Francisco, San Francisco, CA 94143-0738, USA. rajpu@itsa.ucsf.edu

At this time there is no highly sensitive and specific widespread radiographic test for local staging of prostate cancer. Future developments will likely require a combination of imaging modalities with utilization guided by risk-stratification models (Table 4). Staging data for all imaging tests discussed in this article are summarized in Tables 5 and 6. Clinically, conventional gray-scale TRUS remains the most frequently used tool because of its utility in guiding prostatic biopsies. Modifications of TRUS--including power and color Doppler, 3D imaging, and new ultrasound contrast agents and elastography--show promise in increasing the accuracy of ultrasound. Endorectal MRI may have some value for staging selected patients. The addition of prostatic MRS, which images the differential activity of metabolites, may increase the specificity of MRI. Newer techniques with finer voxel resolution may prove to be clinically useful. A large well-designed study evaluating the utility of MRI/MRS is currently being planned. Cross-sectional imaging of the pelvis with either MRI or CT should be used selectively as should radionuclide bone scans. Similarly, ProstaScint scans should be ordered selectively, either before or after primary therapy, rather than routinely in all patients.

3) JS Newman, RL Bree and JM Rubin, Prostate cancer: diagnosis with color Doppler sonography with histologic correlation of each biopsy site. Radiology, Vol 195, 86-90.

Department of Radiology, University of Michigan Hospitals, Ann Arbor, MI 48109-0326.

PURPOSE: To correlate the findings at prostate color Doppler sonography (CDS) with those of site-specific transrectal core biopsy. MATERIALS AND METHODS: Forty-three patients underwent prostate transrectal ultrasonography (US) and biopsy. CDS was performed at all biopsy sites before US-guided core biopsy. Vascularity at CDS was prospectively graded on a scale of 0-2 (0 = no visible peripheral zone [PZ] flow, 2 = markedly increased PZ vascularity). CDS results were correlated with histologic findings from 220 separate biopsy sites that included 27 focal lesions.

RESULTS: Of 34 grade 2 biopsy sites, 21 revealed carcinoma, eight revealed prostatitis, and five were negative. CDS depicted at least one focus of carcinoma in seven patients with no gray- scale abnormality. CDS had a sensitivity of 49%, specificity of 93%, and positive predictive value of 62%.

CONCLUSION: Focal PZ hypervascularity at CDS is associated with an increased likelihood of prostate cancer or inflammation at biopsy, often without a focal gray-scale abnormality. CDS may help identify an appropriate site for biopsy. A negative CDS scan, however, should not preclude biopsy, as CDS has a limited sensitivity in the detection of all sites of cancer.

4) Frauscher F, et al, Ultrasound contrast agents and prostate cancer. Radiologe. 2005 Jun;45(6):544-51. Klinik fur Radiodiagnostik II, Medizinische Universitat Innsbruck.

Prostatic carcinoma is the most frequent malignant disease in men and associated with very high mortality. The diagnostic work-up of prostatic carcinoma is based on tests to determine the level of prostate-specific antigen (PSA), digital rectal examination, and transrectal sonography. Due to diagnostic limitations, ultrasound-guided prostate biopsy is the method of choice for diagnosis of prostatic carcinoma. New imaging technologies allow detection of prostatic carcinoma, thus facilitating removal of specific biopsy specimens from these regions. Introduction of ultrasound contrast agents ("echo signal enhancers") significantly increased the diagnostic potential of this method, making it possible to visualize tumor vascularization.

5) Heijmink SW, van Moerkerk H, Kiemeney LA, Witjes JA, Frauscher F, Barentsz JO, A comparison of the diagnostic performance of systematic versus ultrasound-guided biopsies of prostate cancer. Eur Radiol. 2006 Jan 4: 1-12.

Department of Radiology, Radboud University Nijmegen Medical Centre, Geert Grooteplein zuid 10, 6500 HB, Nijmegen, The Netherlands.

Transrectal ultrasound (TRUS) is an important tool for urologists and radiologists in the detection of prostate cancer. Various TRUS-guided biopsy techniques are applied in clinical practice. Frequently, only the detection rates achieved with these methods are compared. Other diagnostic performance parameters, particularly the specificity and negative predictive value, are seldom compared. After extensive assessment of the available literature, this review describes the methods of TRUS-guided biopsy for prostate cancer detection. A distinction was made between systematic biopsies and biopsies that target a perceived (hypoechoic or Doppler-enhancing) lesion on imaging. Subsequently, the diagnostic performance (sensitivity, specificity, positive and negative predictive values, accuracies) was compared between these techniques. Imaging-guided biopsy showed better diagnostic performance than systematic biopsy with higher sensitivity. The combinations of sensitivity and specificity were highest for colour Doppler and contrast-enhanced targeted biopsy. Studies targeting hypoechoic lesions had relatively high sensitivity, but specificity was low. Presently however, with widespread prostate-specific antigen screening, fewer prostate cancers are hypoechoic, and the value of targeting hypoechoic lesions has diminished. Performing colour or contrast-enhanced Doppler biopsy or adding these techniques to systematic biopsies improves diagnostic performance, particularly by increasing sensitivity.

6) Roy C, Buy X, Lang H, Saussine C, Jacqmin D., Contrast enhanced color Doppler endorectal sonography of prostate: efficiency for detecting peripheral zone tumors and role for biopsy procedure. J Urol. 2003 Jul;170 (1):69-72.

Department of Radiology B, University Hospital of Strasbourg-Hopital Civil, 1 place de l'hopital, 67091 Strasbourg Cedex, France.

PURPOSE: We evaluated the accuracy of contrast enhanced color Doppler endorectal ultrasound to guide biopsy for the detection of prostate cancer.

MATERIALS AND METHODS: A total of 85 patients were evaluated with gray scale and color Doppler before and during intravenous injection of ultrasound contrast agent made of galactose based air microbubbles. Our biopsy protocol was performed during contrast injection. An additional 18 directed cores were obtained based on contrast enhanced imaging. Diagnostic efficiency with and without contrast medium injection for detecting prostate cancer were compared based on biopsy results.

RESULTS: Cancer was identified in a total of 58 biopsy sites in 54 patients. Gray scale imaging revealed 96 abnormal hypoechoic nodules or irregular zones inside the outer gland, of which 48 were malignant on pathological evaluation. Contrast enhanced color Doppler had higher sensitivity (93%) than unenhanced color Doppler (54%), while specificity increased only 79% to 87% for enhanced imaging. Nine of 10 isoechoic suspicious zones were depicted with enhancement, while unenhanced Doppler detected 7 of them. There was no significant difference between the intensity of enhancement and tumor Gleason scores.

CONCLUSIONS: Contrast enhanced color Doppler endorectal sonography increases the detection of prostate cancer. Improvement in sensitivity was high, while the difference in specificity was not as pertinent. It is accurate when using a common and routine application ultrasound unit. This technique is easy to perform and not time-consuming. Obtaining additional biopsy cores of suspicious enhancing foci significantly improves the detection rate of cancer.

7) Sauvain JL, Palascak P, Bourscheid D, Chabi C, Atassi A, Bremon JM, Palascak R, **Value of power Doppler and 3D vascular sonography as a method for diagnosis and staging of prostate cancer.** Eur Urol. 2003 Jul;44(1):21-30; discussion 30-1.

Medical Imaging Center, 6 passage Jules Didier, Vesoul 70000, France.

OBJECTIVES: To compare the value of Power Doppler Sonography (PDS) and B mode sonography in the diagnosis of prostate cancer and to assess the value of PDS to specify capsular effraction of the cancer.

PATIENTS AND METHODS: 323 patients were investigated: 41 control subjects allowed the establishment of normal vascular semiology and 282 patients with suspected cancer (PSA >4ng/ml). Power Doppler Sonography with 3D reconstruction was used to describe Power Doppler Sonography features of normal or abnormal vessels. Three types of blood supply (a: regular avascular posterior peripheral margin, b: irregular avascular posterior peripheral margin, c: vessels crossing the posterior peripheral margin) were described as a function of the presumed stage of cancer (a: intraprostatic, b: undetermined, c: extraprostatic). Comparison with histology was performed on random biopsies without Doppler (282 cases) (median PSA level = 15.8ng/ml), on second biopsies indicated with PDS (72 cases), and radical prostatectomy specimens (63 cases).

RESULTS: A cancer was diagnosed in 157 of the 282 patients (55.7%) with suspected cancer. The overall sensitivity of PDS in the initial diagnosis of prostatic cancer was 92.4% and its specificity was 72% (versus 87.9% and 57.6% for sonography alone respectively). The negative predictive value of PDS was elevated to 80.6% ($p<0.0001$). Targeting area presenting abnormal blood flow in any part of the prostate was useful to detect isoechoic or lesions in patients with first negative biopsy results (in 41 of 72 targeted patients with first negative biopsies with PDS a cancer was diagnosed: 58% of these cancers had less than 3 positive biopsies and 34% only one positive biopsy). The 3 vascular types a, b, c were evaluated prospectively in the detection of capsular effraction. The presence or absence of vessels crossing the capsule to determine an extracapsular extension was a significant sign ($p<0.0001$). Capsular effraction was detected in 3 of the 27 cases (11%) of type a cancer and in 16 of the 18 cases (87%) of type c cancer.

CONCLUSION: PDS improves the accuracy of echographic imaging in the diagnosis of cancer. Combining first sextant biopsies and targeted areas presenting abnormal blood flow using PDS can increase cancer detection with an optimized number of biopsy cores. The risk of extracapsular involvement can be evaluated by the presence of vessels perforating the capsule.

8) Merkle W, Colour Doppler transrectal 3D-sonography of the prostate--first experiences. Aktuelle Urol. 2002 Jan;33(1):53-7.

Fachbereich Urologie, Stiftung Deutsche Klinik fur Diagnostik GmbH, Aukammallee 33, 65191 Wiesbaden.

INTRODUCTION: Early detection of prostate carcinoma still is problematic in spite of advantages in lab testing and sonography. This report demonstrates the new technique of colour Doppler 3-dimensional transrectal ultrasound in differential diagnosis of elevated PSA.

CASE REPORTS: In 13 cases this new ultrasound technique is described and typical results are demonstrated. All cases are histologically and clinically verified.

CONCLUSION: Colour Doppler 3-dimensional transrectal ultrasound is a useful new technique with specific diagnostic capabilities for differential diagnosis of an increased PSA level. Prostate carcinoma can be detected early, prostatitis can be found easily and therapeutic effects can be followed. Colour Doppler 3-dimensional transrectal ultrasound has however to prove in clinical comparative studies its specific advantages for screening of prostate carcinoma.

9) Cheng S, Rifkin MD, Color Doppler imaging of the prostate: important adjunct to endorectal ultrasound of the prostate in the diagnosis of prostate cancer. Ultrasound Q. 2001 Sep;17(3):185-9.

Reston Radiology Associates, Reston, Virginia, USA.

The purpose of this article is to evaluate color Doppler imaging (CDI) as an adjunctive tool to gray-scale ultrasound (US) in the diagnosis of prostate cancer and to correlate CDI-positive lesions to cancer grade. We retrospectively analyzed 619 consecutive patients who underwent prostate US, CDI, and biopsy because of abnormal digital rectal examination results or prostate-specific antigen levels. All had directed (into a specific lesion) biopsies or directed biopsies along with systematic four-quadrant or sextant biopsies, or systematic biopsy alone. Color Doppler imaging was compared with gray-scale findings and histologic results. There were 222 (35.9%) biopsy-proven cancers (n = 197) or prostatic intraepithelial neoplasia (n = 25). Of these, 106 (47.7%) had color-flow abnormalities. Of these 106 patients, 26 (24.5%), or 11.7% of all cancer patients, had relatively normal gray-scale US findings but had focal CDI abnormalities as the method of identification. Overall, 76.9% of these were moderate to high Gleason grades and were considered clinically significant lesions. Color Doppler imaging can identify a large number (11.7%) of clinically significant prostate cancers that are poorly seen by gray-scale US. Positive lesions on CDI are of clinical importance because 76.9% are histologically, moderately, or poorly differentiated. We recommend that CDI be used in all diagnostic and biopsy-guided US examinations of the prostate.

10) Feleppa EJ, Ennis RD, Schiff PB, Wuu CS, Kalisz A, Ketterling J, Urban S, Liu T, Fair WR, Porter CR, Gillespie JR, Ultrasonic spectrum-analysis and neural-net-

work classification as a basis for ultrasonic imaging to target brachytherapy of prostate cancer. Brachytherapy. 2002;1(1):48-53.

Biomedical Engineering Laboratories, Riverside Research Institute, New York, NY 10038, USA.

Conventional B-mode ultrasound is the standard means of imaging the prostate for guiding prostate biopsies and planning brachytherapy of prostate cancer. Yet B-mode images do not allow adequate visualization of cancerous lesions of the prostate. Ultrasonic tissue-typing imaging based on spectrum analysis of radiofrequency echo signals has shown promise for overcoming the limitations of B-mode imaging for visualizing prostate tumors. Tissue typing based on radiofrequency spectrum analysis uses nonlinear methods, such as neural networks, to classify tissue by using spectral-parameter and clinical-variable values. Two- and three-dimensional images based on these methods show potential for improving the guidance of prostate biopsies and the targeting of radiotherapy of prostate cancer. Two-dimensional images have been imported into instrumentation for real-time biopsy guidance and into commercial dose-planning software for brachytherapy planning. Three-dimensional renderings seem to be capable of depicting locations and volumes of cancer foci.

11) Lee F, Bahn DK, Siders DB, Greene C, The role of TRUS-guided biopsies for determination of internal and external spread of prostate cancer. Semin Urol Oncol. 1998 Aug;16(3):129-36.

Department of Radiology, Crittenton Hospital, Ann Arbor, MI 48307, USA.

This study hopes to define local extent of newly diagnosed prostate cancer by comparing sextant biopsies with transrectal ultrasound-guided diagnostic and staging biopsies. The study group consists of 110 men with sextant biopsy proven prostate cancer who presented for an opinion for prognosis and treatment options. All patients were rediagnosed and staged by transrectal ultrasound-guided and staging biopsies. Tumor diagnosis was substantiated in 94.5% (104 of 110). For the 5.4% (6 of 110) not detected by transrectal ultrasonography, review of their outside slides revealed 83.3% (5 of 6) with cancer < or =2 mm with a Gleason score of < or =6. These have the criteria of latent cancers. For the remaining 104 patients with transrectal ultrasound proven cancer, 30% (31 of 104) had extracapsular extension. Sextant and directed biopsy confirmed stage T3 in 3.8% (4 of 104). For clinical stages T1c and T2, 19% and 30%, respectively, had extracapsular extension. Perineural invasion was 1.9 times greater for directed biopsies than sextant biopsies (P < .001. The mean Gleason score was greater for directed biopsies than sextant biopsies, although no statistical difference was found (P > .05). For these 104 patients, 50% (52 of 104) had perineural invasion, of which 38.5% (20 of 52) had proven extracapsular extension. In our hands, transrectal ultrasound-directed and staging biopsies afford more substantive results than sextant biopsies for detecting extracapsular extension. For our cohort of sextant T1-T2 diagnosed cancer (n = 100), 27% were upstaged to T3-T4 by transrectal ultrasound-directed staging biopsy. Thus, transrectal ultrasound-directed staging biopsy has the ability to diagnose unsuspected extracapsular extension and objectifies prognosis and choice of definitive treatment.

Also see: Bahn DK, Color Doppler and Tissue Harmonic Ultrasound in the Early Detection and Staging of Prostate Cancer. Prostate Institute of America, PCRI Insights, Nov. 2002, v5.2. This article is reprinted on the Prostate Cancer Research Institute Web site located at:

www.prostate-cancer.org/education/staging/Bahn_ColorDopplerUltrasound.html

12) Prostate biopsies using both gray scale and 3D color flow power Doppler ultrasound (3DCFPDU)—ASCO 2015 Genitourinary Cancer Symposium—February 26-28, 2015

AUTHORS:

Michael J. Dattoli, MD—Physician-in-Chief
Richard A. Sorace, MD, PhD—Medical Director
    Dattoli Cancer Center & Brachytherapy Research Institute
    Sarasota, Florida

Stephen M. Bravo, MD
    University of Central Florida Assistant Professor
    Orlando, Florida
    Sand Lake Imaging—Founder
    Orlando, Florida

David Bostwick, MD—Founder
    Bostwick Laboratories Richmond, Virginia;
    Orlando, Florida

BACKGROUND: Prostate Cancer (CAP) diagnosis has historically been identified through random biopsies using transrectal ultrasound guided biopsies (TRUS).

Today's standard protocol typically consists of an "extended pattern" 10-12 core biopsy method.

This often leads to sampling errors with mixed diagnosis, delayed diagnosis and the need for repeated biopsies, under staging and finding indolent malignancies leading to over treatment. Infection is not uncommon when using standard TRUS, which is avoided when using sterile transperineal methods.

Advantages in 3D color flow power Doppler ultrasound (3DCFPDU) suggest that more selective biopsies are superior to standard TRUS biopsies, resulting in a higher yield of CAP.

METHODS: 192 consecutive patients were biopsied using 3DCFPD between February 2012 and July 2014. Patients were positioned in the extended dorsolithotomy position allowing maximal visualization of all regions of the prostate regardless of size. Local anesthesia was utilized. The median number of biopsies per patient was eight (8). Only 3 patients had not undergone previous biopsies and median previous biopsies = 2.

We studied tumor detection rate using combined gray scale and 3DCFPDU with directly sampling of specific regions using the transperineal brachytherapy template guided method as a simple outpatient procedure.

Inclusion criteria consisted of abnormal DRE, PSA kinetics 0.75ng/mg/yr, PSA >10 and % free PSA <17, PSA density 0.27. Cores were stratified into 4 risk groups:
1. Hypoechoic only lesion (72 patients, 648 cores)
2. Hypervascular only lesion (26 patients, 182 cores)
3. Hypoechoic lesion associated with hypervascular pulsatile vessels which were synchronous and coinciding with normal cardiac pulse using duplex analysis (32 patients, 256 cores)
4. Hypoechoic lesion associated with non-pulsatile vessels suggesting independent vascular flow consistent with neoplasm also using duplex analysis (62 patients, 434 cores) NOTE: Isoechoic regions were not biopsied. Subgroups were analyzed using chi-square, student t-test and logistic regression.

RESULTS: The diagnosis yield associated with Group 4 was statistically significantly higher compared to:

Risk Group 1. 20% biopsy positive (p <0.5)
Risk Group 2. 19% biopsy positive (p<0.3)
Risk Group 3. 55% biopsy positive (p<0.1)
Risk Group 4. 97% biopsy positive (p<0.01)

Only group 4 revealed a greater Gleason 7-10 CAP (p<0.03).

CONCLUSION: Transperineal template guided biopsies using gray scale and 3DCF-PDU are both highly effective and cost effective.

This may lead to reducing the number of prostate biopsies performed resulting in reduced post-procedure morbidity, more accurate staging while allowing for enhanced detection of serious CAP by targeting the most suspicious lesions.

Additional research should study the diagnostic gain associated with 3DCFPDU.

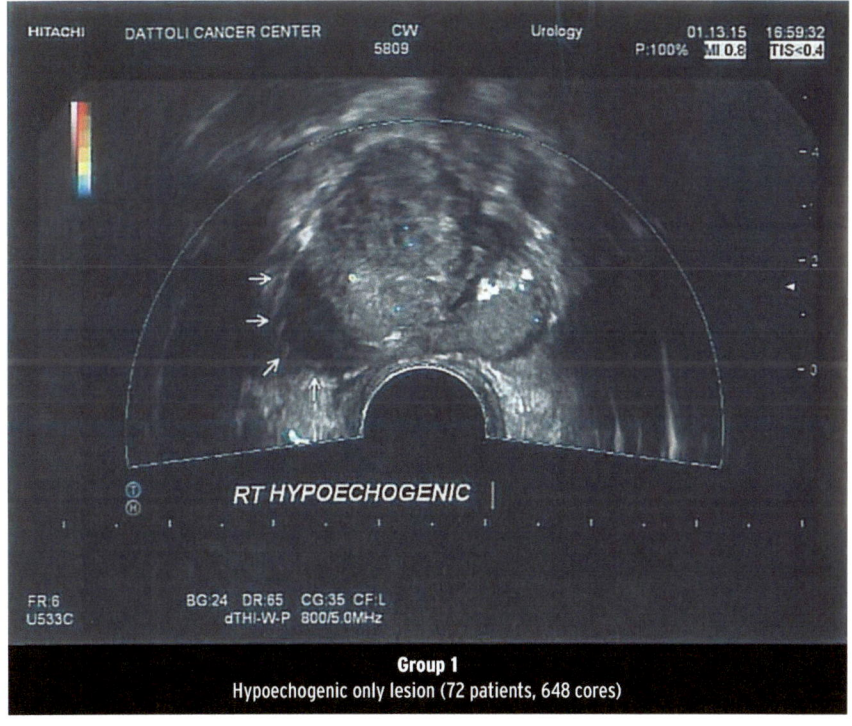

Group 1
Hypoechogenic only lesion (72 patients, 648 cores)

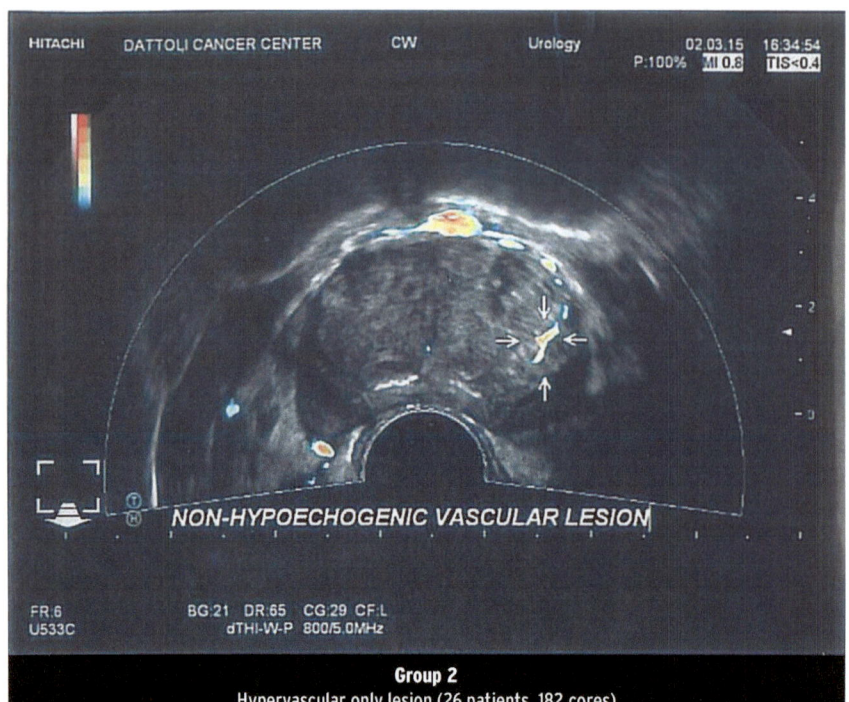

Group 2
Hypervascular only lesion (26 patients, 182 cores)

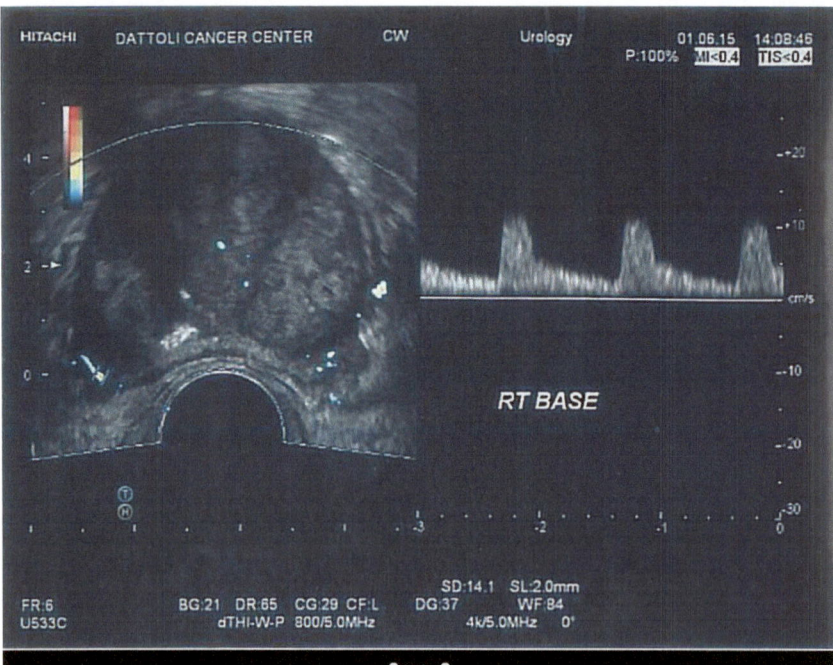

Group 3
Hypoechogenic lesion associated with pulsatile vessels (32 patients, 256 cores)

APPENDIX A: ABSTRACTS AND REFERENCES

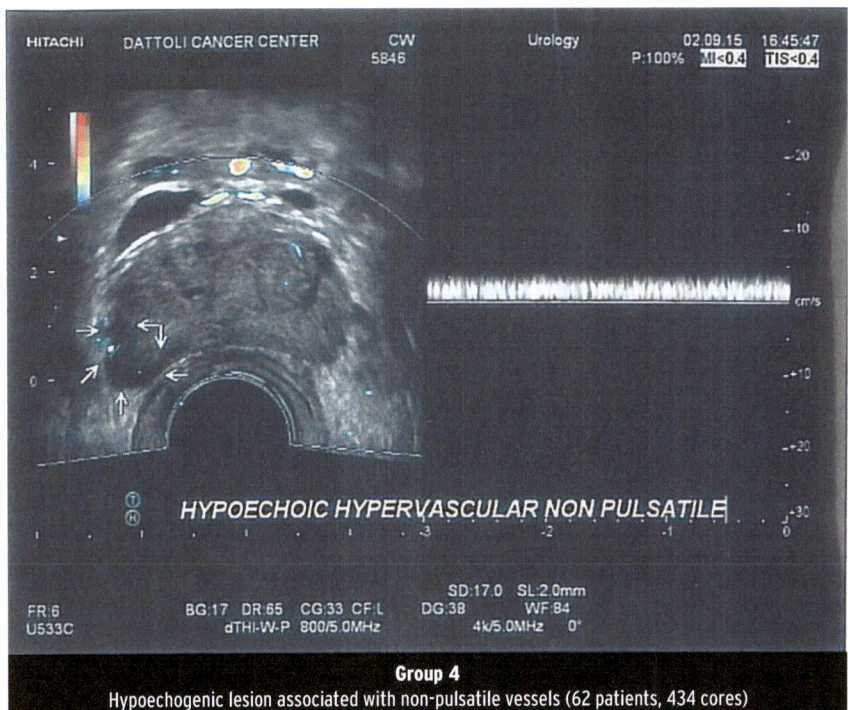

Group 4
Hypoechogenic lesion associated with non-pulsatile vessels (62 patients, 434 cores)

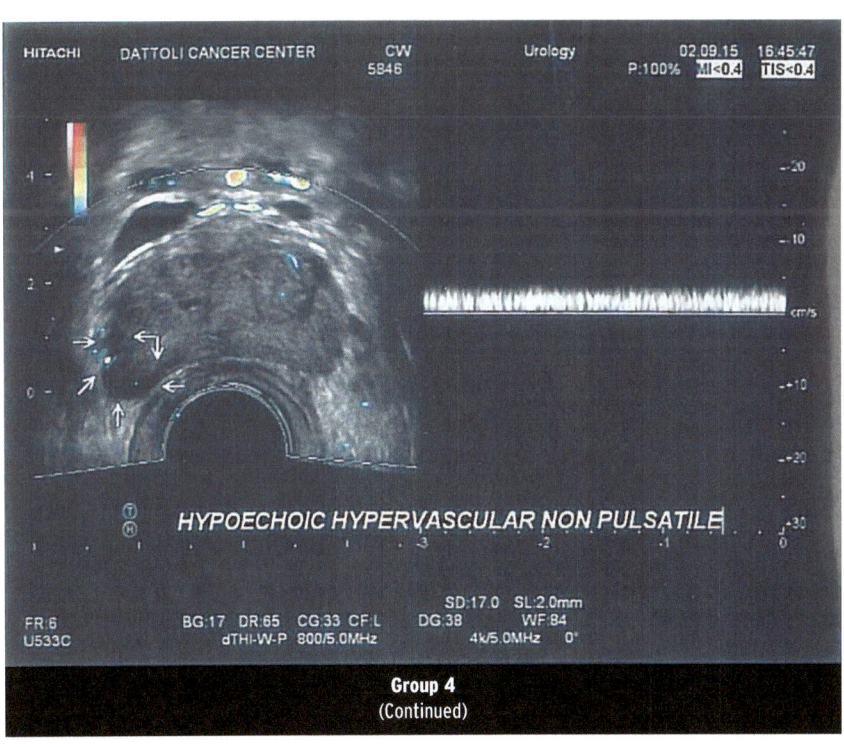

Group 4
(Continued)

13) Our Dattoli Team research with Feraheme-Ferumoxytol was recently confirmed by researchers at the University of Pennsylvania.

REPURPOSING FERUMOXYTOL: Diagnostic and therapeutic applications of an FDA-approved nanoparticle

Yue Huang[1,2,3], Jessica C. Hsu[1,4], Hyun Koo[2,3], David P. Cormode[1,4 Error! Filename not specified].

1. Department of Radiology, Perelman School of Medicine, University of Pennsylvania, Philadelphia, PA, USA
2. Biofilm Research Labs, Levy Center for Oral Health, School of Dental Medicine, University of Pennsylvania, Philadelphia, PA, USA
3. Department of Preventive & Restorative Sciences, School of Dental Medicine, University of Pennsylvania, Philadelphia, PA, USA
4. Department of Bioengineering, School of Engineering and Applied Sciences, University of Pennsylvania, Philadelphia, PA, USA

CITATION: Huang Y, Hsu JC, Koo H, Cormode DP. Repurposing ferumoxytol: Diagnostic and therapeutic applications of an FDA-approved nanoparticle. *Theranostics* 2022; 12(2):796-816. doi:10.7150/thno.67375. Available from https://www.thno.org/v12p0796.htm

ABSTRACT: Ferumoxytol is an intravenous iron oxide nanoparticle formulation that has been approved by the U.S. Food and Drug Administration (FDA) for treating anemia in patients with chronic kidney disease. In recent years, ferumoxytol has also been demonstrated to have potential for many additional biomedical applications due to its excellent inherent physical properties, such as superparamagnetism, biocatalytic activity, and immunomodulatory behavior. With good safety and clearance profiles, ferumoxytol has been extensively utilized in both preclinical and clinical studies. Here, we first introduce the medical needs and the value of current iron oxide nanoparticle formulations in the market. We then focus on ferumoxytol nanoparticles and their physicochemical, diagnostic, and therapeutic properties. We include examples describing their use in various biomedical applications, including magnetic resonance imaging (MRI), multimodality imaging, iron deficiency treatment, immunotherapy, microbial biofilm treatment and drug delivery. Finally, we provide a brief conclusion and offer our perspectives on the current limitations and emerging applications of ferumoxytol in biomedicine. Overall, this review provides a comprehensive summary of the developments of ferumoxytol as an agent with diagnostic, therapeutic, and theranostic functionalities.

INTRODUCTION: Iron oxide nanoparticles have been increasingly used in a variety of biomedical applications because of their inherent multifunctional properties, such as superparamagnetic behavior and biocatalytic activity. These nanoparticles can possess different crystal structures including hematite (α-Fe_2O_3), maghemite (γ-Fe_2O_3), and magnetite (Fe_3O_4). Synthetic control over the particle's composition, size, morphology, and surface chemistry has specific impacts on its biodistribution, pharmacokinetics, and suitability for various biomedical uses. In particular, iron oxide nanoparticles with extremely small core sizes ranging between 3 nm and 15 nm have broad applicability and high translational potential. Nevertheless, iron oxide cores (particularly magnetite) are easily oxidized in air and are insoluble in aqueous solution. Thus, surface coatings that can maintain iron oxide nanoparticle stability in biological media and prevent the loss of magnetism are necessary.

Numerous iron oxide nanoparticle formulations have been studied in both preclinical and clinical settings. Some of these formulations have already appeared on the market. It is estimated that the global market for biomedically applied magnetic particles will reach US $87.7 million by 2025 and will increase by 10% annually. This is largely driven by the growing population of patients with renal diseases as well as increasing demands for the diagnosis and treatment for certain diseases. Therefore, the economic prospects for iron oxide nanoparticles are very good. The following iron oxide nanoparticles have been approved by the U.S. Food and Drug Administration (FDA) for clinical use: Feraheme® for iron deficiency; Combidex® (U.S.) and Sinerem® (Europe) as a magnetic resonance imaging (MRI) agent; Nanotherm® (MagForce) for cancer treatment; and Lumirem® as an oral gastrointestinal tract imaging agent.

Among these iron oxide nanoparticles, Feraheme® (ferumoxytol injectable solution) was approved in the U.S. in 2009, Canada in 2011, and Europe in 2012 and has been used for treating iron-deficiency anemia (IDA), which is often found in renally impaired patients. Moreover, ferumoxytol holds great promise for many other biomedical applications including MRI, drug delivery, oral biofilm treatment, and anti-cancer and anti-inflammatory therapies. Notably, ferumoxytol is being used as an MRI contrast agent in ongoing clinical.

Additional References

Badiozamani et al, Comparability of CT-based and TRUS-based prostate volumes. Int J Radiat Oncol Biol Phys. 1999 Jan 15;43 (2):375-8.

Zaider et al, Treatment planning for prostate implants using magnetic-resonance spectroscopy imaging. Int J Radiat Oncol Biol Phys. 2000 Jul 1;47 (4):1085-96.

Mizowaki, et al, Towards integrating functional imaging in the treatment of prostate cancer with radiation: the registration of the MR spectroscopy imaging to ultrasound/CT images and its implementation in treatment planning. Int J Radiat Oncol Biol Phys. 2002 Dec 1;54 (5):1558-64.

Scheidler J, Hricak H, Vigneron DB, et al, Prostate cancer: localization with three-dimensional proton MR spectroscopic imaging - clinicopathologic study. Radiology 213:473-80, 1999.

Yu KK, Scheidler J, Hricak H, et al: Prostate cancer: prediction of extracapsular extension with endorectal MR imaging and three-dimensional proton MR spectroscopic imaging. Radiology 213:481-8, 1999.

Kurhanewicz J, Vigneron DB, Males RG, et al: The Prostate: Magnetic Resonance Imaging and Spectroscopy: Present and Future. In: Hricak H and Carroll PR, eds. Radiological Clinics of North America. Philadelphia. W.B. Saunders Co., pp. 115-138, 2000.

Barentsz,J, Heesakkers RA, Hovels AM, Jager GJ et al. MRI with a lymph-node-specific contrast agent as an alternative to CT scan and lymphnode dissection in patients with prostate cancer: a prospective multicohort study. Lancet Oncology, 2008.

Bluestein DL, Bostwick DG, Bergstrahlh EJ, Osterling JE. Eliminating the need for bilateral pelvic lymphadenectomy in select patients with prostate cancer. J Urol 1994; 151: 1315-20.

Hövels AM, Heesakkers RA, Adang EM, Barentsz JO, Jager GJ, Severens JL. Cost-effectiveness of MR lymphography for the detection of lymph node metastases in patients with prostate cancer. Radiology. 2009 Sep;252(3):729-36.

Heesakkers RA, Jager GJ, Hövels AM, de Hoop B, van den Bosch HC, Raat F, Witjes JA, Mulders PF, van der Kaa CH, Barentsz JO. Prostate cancer: detection of lymph node metastases outside the routine surgical area with ferumoxtran-10-enhanced MR imaging. Radiology. 2009 May;251(2):408-14.

APPENDIX B

ADVANCED IMAGING AND TREATMENT PLANNING AT THE DATTOLI CANCER CENTER AND BRACHYTHERAPY INSTITUTE

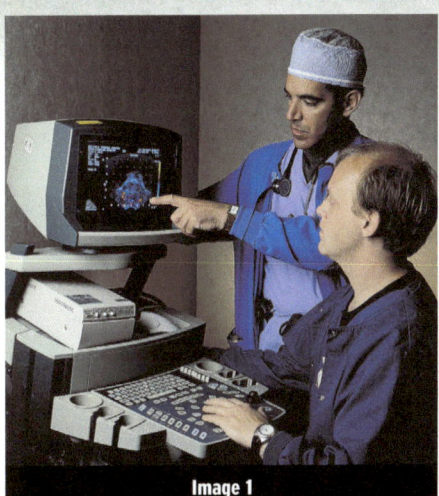

Image 1
3D Color-Flow Power Doppler Ultrasound is used to image cancer areas inside and outside the prostate gland. At our center, patients are invited to view their 3D Color-Flow Power Doppler Ultrasound images in order to visualize the treatment process.

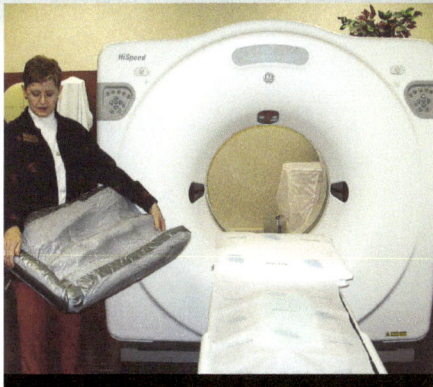

Image 2
The GE High Speed Helical CT Scanner captures high resolution images of the prostate, seminal vesicles, bladder, urethra and rectum, required to accurately design an individual treatment plan. The GE Scanner is also equipped to perform baseline and follow-up QCT Bone Density evaluations. An "alpha cradle" or leg cast, used for immobilization during IMRT treatments, is shown at lower left.

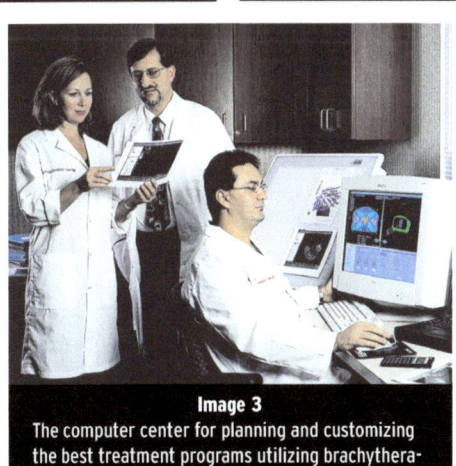

Image 3
The computer center for planning and customizing the best treatment programs utilizing brachytherapy and Image-Guided Intensity Modulated Radiation Therapy (IG-IMRT)

ADVANCED IMAGING FOR PROSTATE CANCER

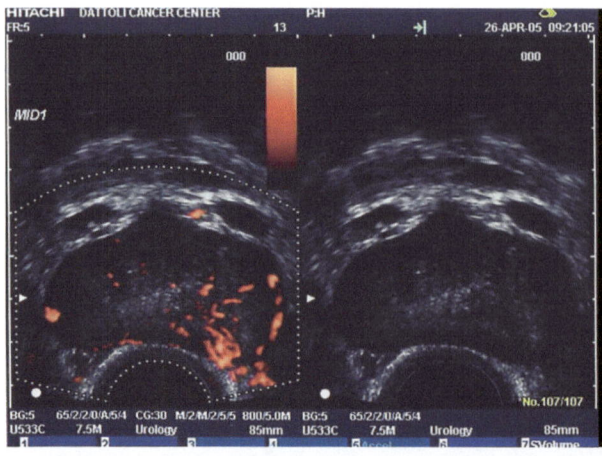

Image 4
A comparison of Color-flow Doppler image (left) with conventional gray-scale ultrasound image (right) of the same patient. The bright red areas in the Color-flow Doppler image reveal the locations of suspected cancer sites which are not visible using gray-scale ultrasound imaging.

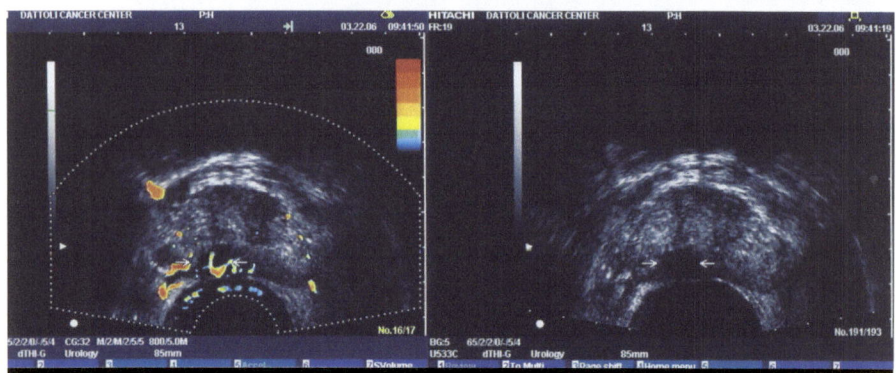

Images 5A and 5B
Another comparison of Color-flow Doppler Image 5A (left) with conventional gray-scale ultrasound Image 5B (right) of the same patient. The two images show the same cross-section of the prostate, with the Color-flow Doppler image revealing the locations of suspected cancer sites in bright red.

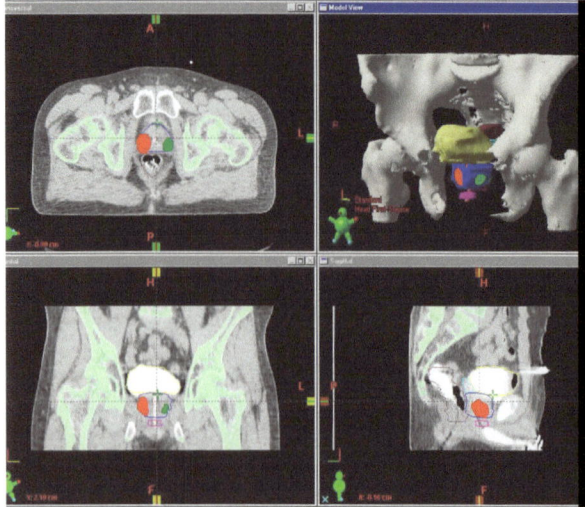

Image 6
Color-flow Doppler abnormalities are fused onto cross-sectional CT scan (upper and lower left, lower right). A special software program then allows the cross-sectional CT scan to be integrated into a 3-dimensional reconstructed model of relevant organs (upper right). Note the organs and structures of interest rendered: bladder is yellow; prostate is blue; penile bulb is purple; urethra is pink; seminal vesicles are light blue; right tumor is red; left tumor is dark green; pelvic bones are light green and white. The very white areas are dense structures such as bone and contrast material.

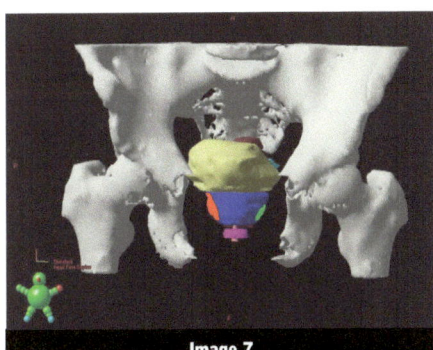

Image 7
Another view of the 3-D image. Bones are white; bladder is yellow; prostate gland is blue; seminal vesicles are light blue; rectum is brown; urethra is pink; penile bulb (where the nerve bundles are located) is purple; right tumor is red; left tumor is dark green.

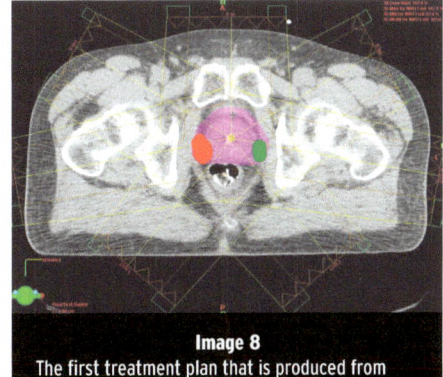

Image 8
The first treatment plan that is produced from the simulation CT scan is called IMRT1, with 7 fields placed in the pattern. The purple area is the volume of interest, which includes the prostate and seminal vesicles.

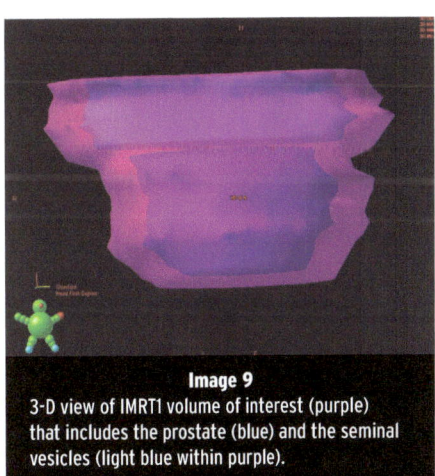

Image 9
3-D view of IMRT1 volume of interest (purple) that includes the prostate (blue) and the seminal vesicles (light blue within purple).

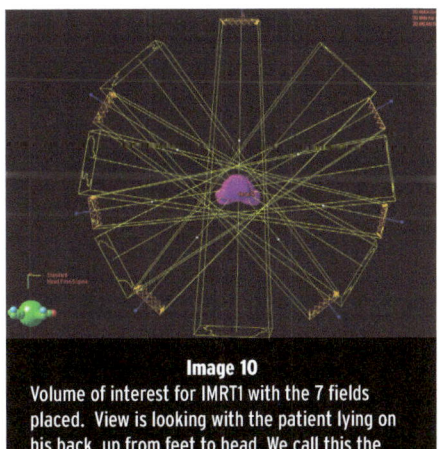

Image 10
Volume of interest for IMRT1 with the 7 fields placed. View is looking with the patient lying on his back, up from feet to head. We call this the "Ferris Wheel."

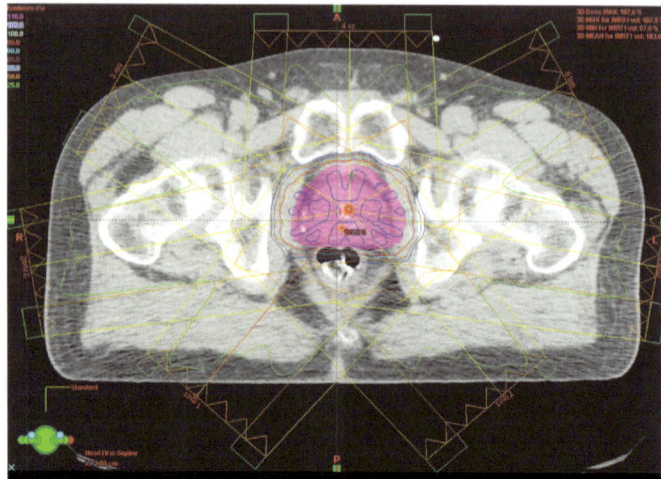

Image 11
We tell the computer what dose we want to direct to the volume of interest and what dose limits we want for the surrounding structures such as the bladder and rectum. The computer gives us the best possible plan which in this view is displayed as isodose lines around the volume of interest. Each line represents a percentage of the dose as outlined in the key in the upper left corner.

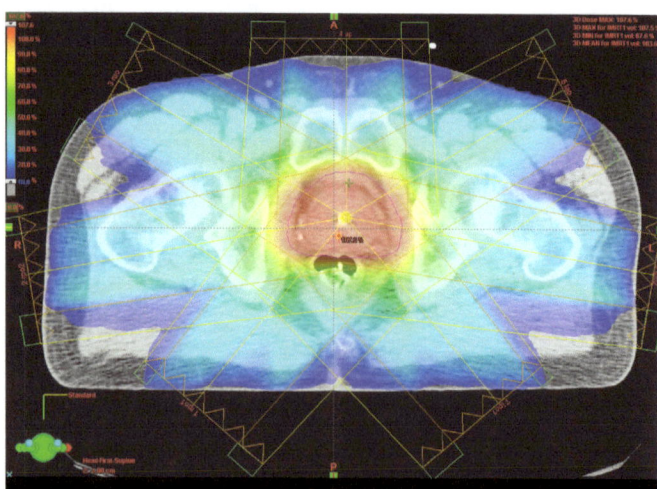

Image 12
This is the same as the previous image but shown in a color wash mode. You can see that where all of the 7 fields converge is where the dose is the "hottest" (color red) and where the dose is "cooler" (color blue). This shows nice uniform coverage around the volume of interest (purple line).

APPENDIX B: ADVANCED IMAGING AND TREATMENT PLANNING AT DATTOLI

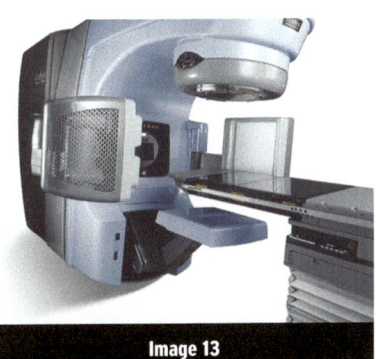

Image 13
A linear accelerator for delivering 4D IG-IMRT with DART, complete with on-board imaging capabilities and the 'exact couch' system.

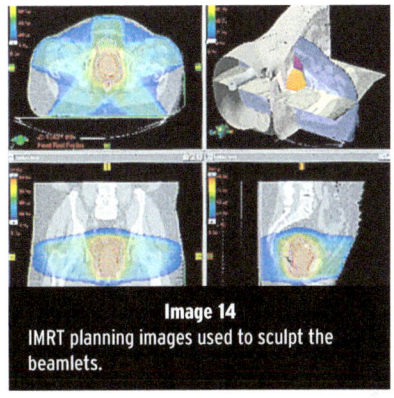

Image 14
IMRT planning images used to sculpt the beamlets.

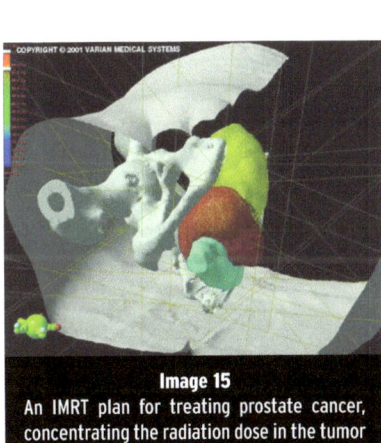

Image 15
An IMRT plan for treating prostate cancer, concentrating the radiation dose in the tumor (red) while avoiding the nearby bladder (yellow) and rectum (green). Courtesy of Varian Medical Systems.

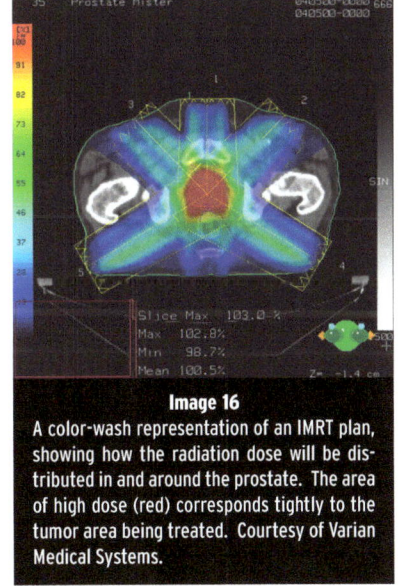

Image 16
A color-wash representation of an IMRT plan, showing how the radiation dose will be distributed in and around the prostate. The area of high dose (red) corresponds tightly to the tumor area being treated. Courtesy of Varian Medical Systems.

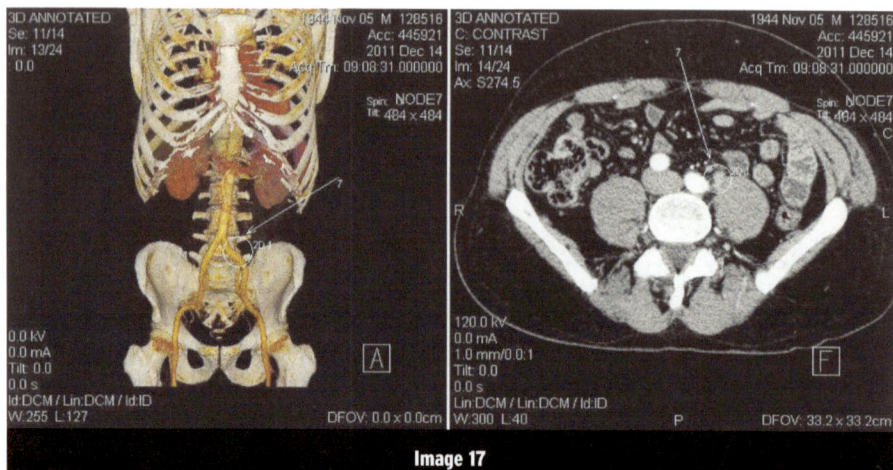

Image 17
A Dynamic Contrast Enhanced MRI study for the identification of cancer metastasis in the lymph nodes.

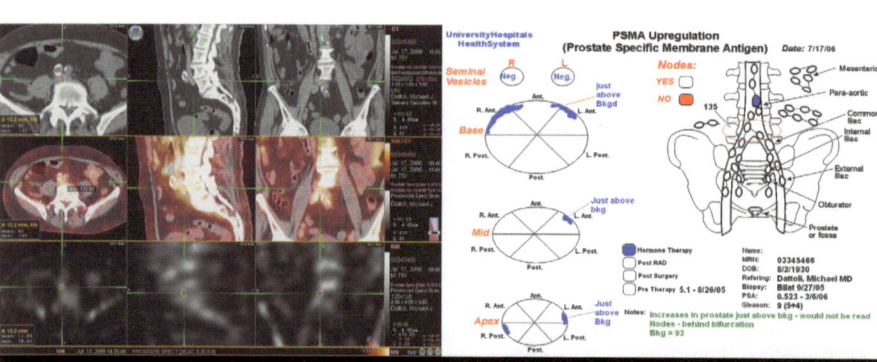

Images 18
ProstaScint® is another diagnostic test that enables doctors to determine lymph node involvement. ProstaScint® can be fused with helical CT or with MRI or with CT/PET scans. A pictorial analysis for this patient appears to the right of the scanned images.

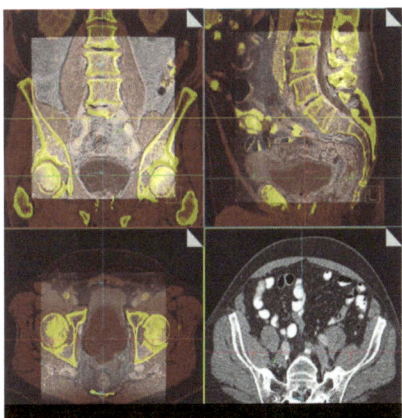

Image 19
The first three images (top right/left and bottom left) are of the abdomen and pelvis in saggital, coronal and axial views. They are MRI fused images that highlight bony anatomy and enhance organs with a rich blood supply. On the first of these images, you can see the right and left kidneys in the upper part of the frame. The last of the four images (bottom right) is a CT scan of the abdomen used to correlate with the fused MRI images for reference.

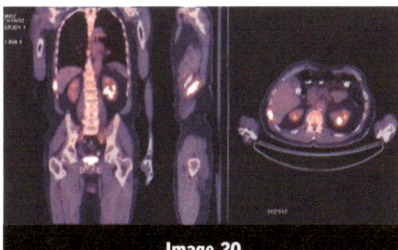

Image 20
The 18F-Fluoride PET/CT imaging technique has demonstrated 100% predictive accuracy (sensitivity and specificity), which is as good as it gets. The images show a biopsy-proven skeletal lesion (metastatic prostate cancer) in one rib, which proved to be treatable. We've pushed the envelope with respect to where we can treat, because the technologies are now so advanced.

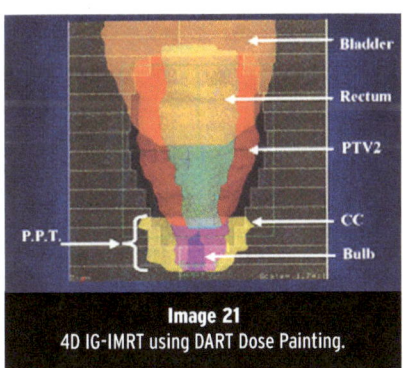

Image 21
4D IG-IMRT using DART Dose Painting.

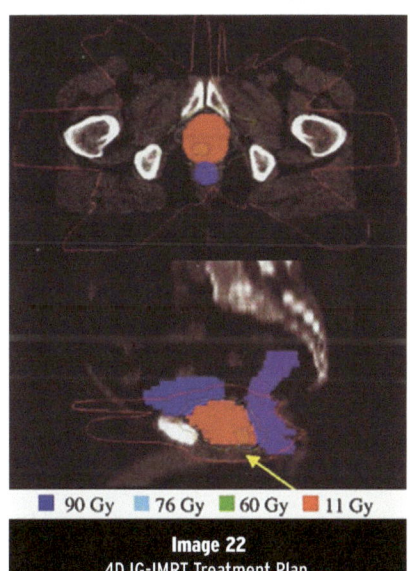

Image 22
4D IG-IMRT Treatment Plan.

APPENDIX C

DECIDING WHAT IS BEST FOR YOU

Consult with your physician, and by all means, obtain second and third opinions whenever possible, preferably from physicians with different specialties. If you have already been to a urologist, it is worthwhile to visit a radiation oncologist or medical oncologist (those with experience with hormones and chemotherapy).

Join a support group such as US TOO!, or PAACT. If you belong to any of the computer on-line services, check out the medical and health bulletin boards and mailing lists for the latest information and announcements for prostate cancer patients. Keep your personal plan of action updated.

What to Remember

- Obtain all of the advice and counsel that you can, but keep in mind that the decisions are ultimately yours to make.

- Be positive—if you have been properly staged and treated, the odds are in your favor on not having a recurrence.

- If you should have a rising PSA over time after initial treatment, don't panic. Get further tests, and if appropriate, get a biopsy, preferably guided by 3D Color-Flow Power Doppler Ultrasound.

- The secret to success with prostate cancer is catching the disease early, and that is also true for recurrence.

- If testing confirms cancer, learn all you can about your options. Get second and third opinions. Become informed and empowered. Become involved with solving your problem. It's your life and body. Go for it!

- Life is full of problems and challenges. Solve this problem like any other big problem:
    1. Identify the problem.
    2. Get all the facts to confirm that you have a problem.
    3. Learn what options are available to you and weigh them carefully.
    4. Choose a qualified doctor who is experienced and with whom you are comfortable.
    5. Initiate and follow through with the solution.
- Don't be afraid to ask for help from your spouse or partner, from your family and your friends. It is more important than ever for you to turn to loved ones to get the emotional and spiritual support you need. This disease can be a difficult struggle for us, but we are not alone, and our mental attitude, prayers and our fighting spirit really can make all the difference.

To be a cancer survivor, you must first be a cancer fighter!

APPENDIX D

GLOSSARY OF MEDICAL TERMS

3D-CRT (3-Dimensional Conformal Radiation Therapy): See Conformal Radiotherapy.

5-alpha reductase (5-AR): an enzyme that converts testosterone to dihydrotestosterone (DHT).

Adenocarcinoma: A cancer originating in glandular tissue. Prostate cancer is classified as adenocarcinoma of the prostate.

Adjuvant: An additional treatment used to increase the effectiveness of the primary therapy. Radiation therapy and hormonal therapy are often used as adjuvant treatments following a radical prostatectomy. Compare Neoadjuvant.

Agonist: A chemical substance that combines with a receptor on a cell and initiates an activity or reaction. See LHRH analogs.

Algorithm: A step-by-step procedure for solving a problem or accomplishing some end, especially by a computer.

Analog: A man-made chemical compound that is structurally similar to one produced naturally by the body. See LHRH analogs.

Anastomotic stricture: *narrowing, usually by scarring, of an anastomotic suture line.*

Androgen: A hormone that produces male characteristics. See testosterone.

Androgen ablation therapy: A therapy designed to inhibit the body's production of testosterones.

Androgen-dependent cells: Prostate cancer cells which are nourished by male hormones and therefore are capable of being destroyed by hormone deprivation (also known as androgen-sensitive cells).

Androgen-independent cells: Prostate cancer cells which are not dependent on male hormones and therefore do not respond to hormonal therapy (also known as androgen-insensitive cells).

Anesthetic: A drug that produces general or local loss of physical sensations, particularly pain. A "spinal" is the injection of a local anesthetic into the area surrounding the spinal cord.

Aneuploid: Having an abnormal number of chromosomes, as revealed by ploidy analysis. Aneuploid prostate cancer cells tend not to respond well to androgen deprivation therapy (ADT).

Angiogenesis: The body's formation of new blood vessels. Some anti-cancer drugs work by blocking angiogenesis, thus preventing blood from reaching and nourishing a tumor.

Antagonist: A chemical substance in the body that acts to reduce the physiological activity of another chemical substance.

Anti-androgens: Drugs such as Casodex that block the activity of androgens produced by the adrenal glands at the cellular receptor sites. Androgens can block or neutralize the effects of testosterone and DHT on prostate cancer cells.

Antibody: A protein produced by the body that counteracts the toxic effects of a foreign substance, organism, or disease within the body.

Antigen: A foreign substance such as a virus or bacterium that causes an immune response or the formation of an antibody.

Antioxidants: Any substances which delay the process of oxidation in the body.

Apoptosis: The normal molecular mechanism which governs the life span of cells so that they die in a very organized way. Cancerous cells are resistant to normal apoptosis.

Benign: A non-cancerous condition. See also Benign Prostatic Hypertrophy.

Benign Prostatic Hypertrophy (BPH): Also called Benign Prostatic Hyperplasia, BPH is a non-cancerous condition of the prostate that results in a growth of tumorous tissue and increase in the size of the prostate.

Biopsy: A procedure involving the removal of tissue from the body of the patient. Removed tissue is typically examined microscopically by a pathologist in order to make a precise diagnosis of the patient's condition.

Bone scan: An imaging technique used to detect bone metastases, which appear as "hot spots" on the film. It is far more sensitive than the conventional x-ray.

BPH: See Benign Prostatic Hypertrophy.

Brachytherapy: A form of radiation therapy in which radioactive seeds are implanted into the prostate to deliver radiation directly to the tumor. Also referred to as seed implantation, or seeding.

APPENDIX D: GLOSSARY OF MEDICAL TERMS

Cancer: A cellular malignancy typically forming tumors. Unlike benign tumors, these tend to invade surrounding tissues and spread to distant sites of the body.

Carcinoma: A malignant tumor made up chiefly of epithelial cells, or those cells that form the lining of an organ or cavity. See Adenocarcinoma.

Castrate Range: The level of the body's testosterone after orchiectomy (also referred to as castration). This is the range or level, which is used by physicians as a point of comparison for those drugs, which attempt to decrease the testosterone level.

CAT Scan (or CT Scan): See Computer Tomography.

cGy: Abbreviation for centigray; a unit of radiation equivalent to the older unit called a "rad."

Chemotherapy: The treatment of cancer using chemicals that deter the growth of cancer cells.

Collimator: A device that organizes radiation such that only parallel rays or beams emanate.

Combination Hormonal Therapy (CHT): Also referred to as Combined Hormonal Blockade (CHB), or Combined Androgen Deprivation Therapy (ADT). The preferred term is ADT, often designated with a number referring to the number of agents used (i.e., monotherapy ADT, ADT2, ADT3). This combined therapy can utilize a number of mechanisms, including surgical or medical ADT, anti-androgens, 5-alpha reductase inhibitors, estrogenic compounds, agents that block adrenal androgen production, and agents that decrease the receptivity of the androgen receptor.

Combination Therapy: Refers generally to any combination of treatment modalities used to treat prostate cancer.

Computer Tomography: Computer generated cross-sectional images of a portion of the body. Also called CT or CAT scan.

Conformal Radiotherapy: A radiation treatment conforming precisely to the size and shape of the prostate, with the use of computerized planning and state-of-the-art imaging techniques. 3-Dimensional Conformal Radiation Therapy (3D-CRT) utilizes this sophisticated approach to treatment planning, as does the even more advanced Intensity Modulated Radiation Therapy (IMRT).

Cryosurgery (also referred to as Cryotherapy or Cryoablation): The freezing of tissue with the use of liquid nitrogen or Argon gas probes. When used to treat prostate cancer, the cryoprobes are guided by transrectal ultrasound.

Cytokine: Any of a class of immunoregulatory substances that are secreted by cells of the immune system.

DHT (dihydrotestosterone): The active form of the male hormone, testosterone, produced after testosterone is transformed by an enzyme known as 5-alpha reductase.

Diagnosis: Evaluation of a patient's symptoms and/or test results, with the intent of identifying and verifying the existence of any underlying disease or abnormal condition.

Digital Rectal Examination (DRE): A procedure in which the physician inserts a gloved, lubricated finger into the rectum to examine the prostate gland for signs of cancer.

DNA (Deoxyribonucleic Acid): A complex protein that is the carrier of genetic information that determines the physical development and growth of living organisms.

Doppler Ultrasound Technique: A machine that sends out ultrasonic waves that pick up the velocity of blood flow through the veins and are transmitted as sound to make an image. The most sophisticated form of this imaging modality is 3D Color-Flow Power Doppler Ultrasound.

Doubling Time: The time it takes for a tumor or cancerous focus to double in size.

Downsizing: The use of hormonal therapy or other forms of intervention to reduce tumor volume prior to primary, curative treatment.

Downstaging: The use of hormonal therapy or other forms of intervention to lower the clinical stage of prostate cancer prior to primary, curative treatment.

Ejaculatory Ducts: The tubular passages through which semen reaches the prostatic urethra during orgasm.

Ejaculation: The release of semen through the penis during orgasm.

Endorectal MRI: Magnetic resonance imaging of the prostate gland using a probe inserted into the rectum. Dynamic Contrast Enhanced MRI is the most effective form of magnetic resonance imaging.

Enzyme: A chemical substance produced by living cells that causes chemical reactions to take place while not being changed itself.

Erectile Dysfunction (also referred to as ED or impotence): The loss of ability to produce and/or sustain an erection sufficient for intercourse.

Estrogen: A female sex hormone that can be used as a form of therapy to inhibit the production of testosterone in patients diagnosed with prostate. cancer.

External Beam Radiation Therapy (EBRT): A form of radiation therapy that utilizes radiation delivered by an external source (machine) and directed at a target area to be radiated. In contrast to EBRT, brachytherapy utilizes radiation sources (seeds) that are internal, implanted in the target tissue. EBRT may use conventional photons, protons, neutrons or electrons.

Extracapsular Extension: Used to describe prostate cancer that has spread outside the prostate gland.

False Negative: An erroneous negative test result. For example, an imaging test that fails to show the presence of a cancer tumor later found by biopsy to be present in the patient is said to have returned a false negative result.

False Positive: A positive test result that mistakenly identifies a state or condition that does not in fact exist.

Feraheme (Ferumoxytol): A ferromagnetic nanoparticle which is taken up by normal macrophages with the lymph nodes.

Fistula: With regard to prostate cancer, an abnormal passage due to injury or disease that connects an abscess or hollow organ to the surface of the body or to another hollow organ. If there is significant damage to the rectal wall proximate to the bladder, a fistula may occur between the bladder and rectum.

Flare Reaction: A testosterone surge caused by the initial use of an LHRH analog, causing a temporary increase of tumor growth and symptoms (known as clinical flare), or an increase in PSA (biochemical flare).

Foley Catheter: A catheter inserted in the penis and threaded through the urethra to the bladder where it is held in place with a tiny, inflated balloon. It removes urine from the bladder and can be used to irrigate the urethra and prevent blood clots.

Free PSA: PSA that is unattached to any major protein in the blood. Free PSA is associated with benign prostate growth. The percentage of free PSA is derived by dividing the free-PSA level by the total-PSA x 100. Studies have show that men with free PSA % > 25% were at low risk for prostate cancer, while men with PSA % < 10% were at high risk for having prostate cancer.

Frozen Section: A technique in which removed tissue is frozen, cut into thin slices, and stained for microscopic examination. A pathologist can rapidly complete a frozen section analysis, and for this reason, it is commonly used during surgery to quickly provide the surgeon with vital information.

Gland: An aggregation of cells (a structure or organ) that secretes a substance for use or discharge from the body.

Gland Volume: The size in cubic centimeters (cc) or grams of the prostate gland.

Gleason Score: A widely used method for classifying the cellular differentiation of cancerous tissue. The less the cancerous cells appear like normal cells, the more malignant the cancer. Two grades of 1-5, identifying the two most common degrees of differentiation present in the examined tissue sample, are added together to produce the Gleason score. High numbers indicate greater differentiation and more aggressive cancer. The grading system is named after its originator, Donald Gleason, M.D.

Globulin: Any of a number of simple proteins that occur widely in plant and animal tissues.

Gynecomastia: A side effect involving breast enlargement and tenderness, associated with various hormonal therapies that increase the level of estrogens in the body.

HDR brachytherapy: High Dose Rate brachytherapy involves the temporary insertion of radioactive iridium isotopes into the prostate gland using transrectal ultrasound guidance.

Hematuria: Blood in the urine.

Hereditary: Inherited genetically from parents and earlier generations.

Holistic Medicine: Medical care, which considers the patient as a whole, including his or her physical, mental, emotional, spiritual, social and economic needs.

Hormone: A substance produced by one tissue or gland and transported by the bloodstream to another to effect or regulate physiological activity such as metabolism and growth.

Hormonal therapy: Cancer treatment involving the blockage of hormone production by surgical or chemical means. Because prostate cancer is usually dependent on male hormones to grow, hormonal therapy can be an effective means of alleviating symptoms and retarding the development of the disease.

Hormone refractory prostate cancer: Prostate cancer that is androgen independent, and therefore, unresponsive to hormonal therapies.

Hot Flash: A side effect of some forms of hormonal therapy, experienced as a sudden rush of warmth to the face, neck, and upper body.

Imaging: Radiology techniques that are often computer-enhanced and allow the physician to visualize areas inside the body that would not normally be visible.

Impotence: See Erectile Dysfunction.

Incontinence: A loss of urinary control. There are various kinds and degrees of incontinence. Overflow incontinence is a condition in which the bladder retains urine after voiding. As a consequence, the bladder remains full most of the time, resulting in involuntary seepage of urine from the bladder. Stress incontinence is the involuntary discharge of urine when there is increased pressure upon the bladder, as in coughing or straining to lift heavy objects. Total incontinence is the failure of ability to voluntarily exercise control over the sphincters of the bladder neck and urethra, resulting in total loss of retentive ability.

Inflammation: Redness or swelling caused by injury or infection.

Informed Consent: Permission to proceed given by a patient after being fully informed of the purposes and potential consequences of a medical procedure.

Intensity Modulated Radiation Therapy (IMRT): The most recent state-of-the-art, computer-aided technique for delivering higher doses of radiation more accurately than either conventional External Beam Radiation or Conformal Radiation. The most advanced form of IMRT is Dynamic Adaptive Radiotherapy (DART).

Intermittent Androgen Deprivation (IAD): A temporary discontinuation of hormonal therapy that allows for a return to natural testosterone production in order to spare the patient from symptoms associated with androgen deprivation. Also referred to as Intermittent Hormonal Therapy (IHT).

Intravenous Pyelogram (IVP): A test that utilizes the injection of a special dye to check for injury or the spread of cancer to the kidneys and bladder.

Investigational: A drug or procedure allowed by the FDA for use in clinical trails, but not necessarily reimbursed.

Isodose Line: A line or two-dimensional shape that circumscribes an area receiving a radiation dose greater than or equal to a specified amount.

Laparoscopic Lymphadenectomy: The removal of pelvic lymph nodes with a laparoscope via four small incisions in the lower abdomen.

LH (Luteinizing Hormone): A chemical signal originating in the pituitary gland that causes the testes to make testosterone.

LHRH Analogs (or LHRH Agonists): Synthetic compounds that are chemically similar to Luteinizing Hormone Releasing Hormone (LHRH), used to suppress testicular production of testosterone. The most commonly prescribed LHRH analogs are Lupron® and Zoldex® Eligard® and Trelstar®. See also Luteinizing Hormone-Releasing Hormone (LHRH).

LHRH Antagonist: A chemical agent that blocks the LHRH receptor without the testosterone surge associated with

LHRH analogs. LHRH antagonists include Abarelix (Plenaxis®).

Linear Accelerator: A high energy x-ray machine generating radiation fields for external beam radiation therapy. These machines are typically mounted with a collimator (or multileaf collimator) in a gantry that rotates vertically around the patient being treated.

Localized Prostate Cancer: Cancer that is confined to the prostate gland, and therefore, considered curable.

Luteinizing Hormone-Releasing Hormone (LHRH): A chemical signal originating in the hypothalamus that causes the pituitary to make LH, which in turn stimulates the testicles to make testosterone.

Lymphadenectomy: The removal and examination of lymph nodes to precisely diagnose and stage cancer. See also Laparascopic Lymphadenectomy.

Lymph Node: A small, bean-shaped mass of tissue located throughout the body along the vessels of the lymphatic system. The lymph nodes filter out bacteria and other toxins, as well as cancer cells.

Magnetic Resonance Imaging (MRI): A painless, non-invasive technique using strong magnetic fields to produce detailed images of internal body structures. An MRI scan usually takes about 45 minutes per site.

Malignancy: A tumorous growth of cancer cells.

Malignant: Having the invasive and metastatic properties of cancer. Tending to become progressively worse and to result in death.

Margin: See Surgical Margin.

Metalloprotease Inhibitors: Drugs used to suppress the body's production of certain enzymes.

Metastasis: The spread of cancer, by way of the blood stream or lymphatic system, beyond the boundaries of the organ or structure where the cancer originated. Metastases is the plural. Metastatic refers to the characteristics associated with cancer that has spread or a secondary tumor.

Metastatic Work-Up: A group of tests, including bone scans, x-rays, and blood tests, to ascertain whether cancer has metastasized.

Monoclonal Antibody (mAb): An antibody that is directed against one specific protein (antigen).

Morbidity: Unhealthy consequences and complications resulting from treatment.

MRI: See Magnetic Resonance Imaging.

Nadir: The lowest point. Doctors sometimes use this as a verb to describe return of cancer or treatment failure. The PSA nadir refers to a minimum PSA value that should be maintained after treatment if the cancer has been successfully eradicated.

Necrosis: Death of cells or tissues caused by disease or injury.

Neoadjuvant: The use of a different type of therapy before primary, curative treatment. For example, neoadjuvant Androgen Deprivation Therapy is often used prior to radiation therapy or radical surgery, with the intent of improving the effectiveness of the primary treatment by reducing the size of the tumor and/or prostate gland.

Nerve-sparing: A procedure used during radical prostatectomy in which the surgeon attempts to save the nerves (neurovascular bundles) that allow for normal sexual functions.

Neurovascular Bundles: Strands of interwoven nerves and veins that run down the side of the prostate. The bundles contain microscopic nerves that are essential for erection; they also contain arteries and veins. Cutting the nerves in the bundles during surgery, or otherwise harming them in another procedure, usually renders the patient impotent.

Nocturia: Getting up at night to urinate.

Non-invasive: Not involving any incision in the body.

Oncogenes: Genes associated with tumor growth.

Oncology: The branch of medical science dealing with tumors. A medical oncologist is a specialist in the study of cancerous tumors.

Organ-confined Disease (OCD): Prostate cancer that is confined to the prostate capsule, as indicated clinically or pathologically.

Orchiectomy: A simple operation that involves surgical removal of the testicles, which produce most of the body's testosterone.

Osteoporosis: A decrease in bone mass and density causing fragility and porosity.

Overstaging: An assessment of an overly high clinical stage at initial diagnosis.

Palpable: Capable of being felt when examined by touch or manipulation.

PAP: See Prostatic Acid Phosphatase.

Pathologist: A doctor who specializes in the examination of cells and tissues removed from the body.

PBRT: See Proton Beam Radiation Therapy.

Perineum: The area of the body between the anus and scrotum. A perineal procedure uses this area as the point of entry into the body.

Perineural Invasion: Describing cancer, which has spread from the prostate to the nerve bundles.

Periprostatic: Relating to the soft tissues immediately proximate to the prostate gland.

Photon: The quantum of electromagnetic energy, described as having zero mass and no electric charge. X-rays are high energy photons.

Placebo: A sugar pill often taken by participants in a medical study. Patients taking a placebo are compared to patients taking actual medications.

Ploidy Analysis: A pathological analysis to determine the number of sets of chromosomes in a cell.

Proctitis: Inflammation of the rectum.

Prognosis: A forecast of the course of a disease and future prospects of the patient.

Progression: A change in the status of the cancer indicating the condition has progressed and worsened.

Pro-oxidant: A term to describe substances that aid in oxidation.

ProstaScint® Scan: An imaging technique sometimes used determine whether or not cancer has spread to distant sites by using monoclonal antibodies.

Prostate Capsule: The outer membranous covering of the prostate gland.

Prostatectomy: The surgical removal of part or all of the prostate gland.

Prostate Specific Antigen (PSA): A blood test that measures a substance manufactured solely by prostate gland cells. An elevated reading indicates an abnormal condition of the prostate gland, either benign or malignant. It is presently the most sensitive tumor marker for the identification and monitoring of prostate cancer.

Prostatic Acid Phosphatase (PAP): An enzyme produced by the prostate that is elevated (3.0 or higher) in many patients when prostate cancer has spread beyond the prostate.

Prostatitis: An infection or inflammation of the prostate gland that is treatable with medications.

Proton Beam Radiation Therapy (PBRT): A form of radiation therapy that utilizes protons as the source of energy (as opposed to X-rays or neutrons).

PSA: See Prostate Specific Antigen.

PSA Bounce (or PSA Bump): A rise in PSA level after first having a reduction in PSA after radiation therapy.

PSA Nadir: The lowest PSA value after a particular treatment.

PSA Velocity (PSAV): The rate of increase of the PSA level, expressed as nanograms per milliliter per year.

Radiation Therapy (RT): The use of high energy rays to kill cancer cells and malignant tissue.

Radiation Urethritis: Inflammation of the urethra caused by radiation therapy.

Radical Prostatectomy: An operation to remove the entire prostate gland and seminal vesicles.

Radiosensitivity: The degree to which a type of cancer responds to radiation therapy.

RBA or Relative Biological Effectiveness: A scale used to compare the intensity of radiation associated with various atomic particles.

Receptor: A cellular docking site that interacts with a specific protein or enzyme (called a ligand). The interaction typically leads to the synthesis of other substances such as proteins, hormones or enzymes.

Recurrence: Return of the cancer following remission or treatment intended as curative. Local recurrence indicates a return of the cancer at the site of origin. Distant recurrence indicates the appearance of one or more metastases of the disease.

Refractory: A term indicating that the cancer no longer responds to the current therapy.

Remission: Complete or partial disappearance of the signs and symptoms of the disease. The period during which a disease remains under control, without progressing. Even complete remission does not necessarily indicate cure.

Resection: The surgical removal of a part of an organ or structure.

Risk: The probability that a particular even will or will not happen.

RP: See Radical Prostatectomy.

RT: See Radiation Therapy.

Rx: The standard abbreviation for prescription.

Salvage Treatment: A medical term for "Plan B." It means a patient must undergo another form of treatment because the first therapy was not successful. Salvage therapy may incur a higher rate of side effects.

Saw Palmetto: A nutrient extracted from the saw palmetto shrub, which is considered by some to aid the body's immune system.

Seed Implantation (SI): A minimally invasive procedure by which radioactive seeds are implanted into the prostate gland to destroy cancer. Also referred to as seeding and brachytherapy.

Selenium: A non-metallic element thought to be beneficial as a nutrient; it is often included in multivitamin supplements.

Seminal Vesicles: Glands that, like the prostate, support male reproduction.

Fluid secreted by these glands regulates the consistency of semen.

Side Effect: A reaction to a treatment or medication, usually referring to an undesirable effect.

Sphincter: A circular muscle which contracts to close an orifice. The urethral sphincter squeezes the urethra shut, providing urinary control.

Staging: The testing process by which the extent and severity of a known cancer is evaluated according to an established system of classification. It is used to help determine appropriate therapy. See TNM Staging and Whitmore-Jewett Staging.

Surgical Margin: The outer edge of the tissue removed during a radical prostatectomy. The surgical margin may be "negative," indicating that no cancer is present and a better prognosis, or "positive," indicating that not all of the cancer has been removed.

Systemic: Throughout the body and affecting the entire body.

T-Cell: An immune system cell or lymphocyte that directs an immune response to malignant or infected cells.

Testes: Two male reproductive glands located inside the scrotum. The testes are the primary sources for testosterone. Also called testicles.

Testosterone: A male sex hormone chiefly produced by the testicles.

Thrombotic: Causing or relating to blood clotting.

TNM Staging: The most widely used classification system for evaluating the extent of prostate cancer. TNM refers to tumor, nodes and metastases. See Staging.

Transrectal: Through the rectum.

Transurethral: Through the urethra.

Transrectal Ultrasonography: See Ultrasound.

Transurethral Resection of the Prostate (TURP): A surgical procedure to remove tissue obstructing the urethra. The technique involves the insertion of an instrument called a resectoscope into the penile urethra, and is intended to relieve obstruction of urine flow due to enlargement of the prostate.

Tumor: An excessive growth of cells that is caused by uncontrolled and disorderly cell replacement. Abnormal tissue growth may be benign or malignant. See also Benign, Malignant.

TURP: See Transurethral Resection of the Prostate.

Ultrasound (Transrectal Ultrasonography): A painless, non-invasive diagnostic imaging technique using sound waves to create an echo pattern that reveals the structure of organs and tissues. It does not use x-rays.

Understaging: An overly low assessment of clinical stage at diagnosis.

Urethra: The tube that carries urine from the bladder and semen from the prostate out of the body through the penis.

Urologist: A physician who specializes in the diagnosis and the medical and surgical treatment of problems in the urinary and male reproductive systems.

USPIO: This technology uses ultrasmall superparamagnetic iron oxide (USPIO) as an MRI contrast agent for the identification of cancer metastasis in lymph nodes.

Vasectomy: A surgical procedure to render a man sterile by cutting the vas deferens, thus eliminating the passage of sperm from the testes to the prostate.

Vasoactive: Causing the dilation or constriction of blood vessels.

Vesicle: A small sac containing fluid, as in seminal vesicles.

Whitmore-Jewett Staging: A classification system for evaluating the extent of prostate cancer. This system is less widely used for the designation of stage than is TNM staging.

X-rays: High energy radiation that can be used at low levels of intensity to make images of the body's internal structures, or at high intensity for radiation therapy.

APPENDIX E

THE WARNING SIGNS OF PROSTATE CANCER

There are often no warning signs of prostate cancer. In some cases the following symptoms may indicate the presence of the disease. However, please be aware that these symptoms may also be due to benign conditions of the prostate, or other conditions entirely unrelated to prostate cancer:

- Elevated or rising PSA
- Abnormal Digital Rectal Exam
- Blood in urine
- Pain or difficulty urinating
- Increased urge to urinate, especially at night
- Hesitant or intermittent urinary flow
- Pain or discomfort in area of prostate
- Unusual and unexplained weight loss
- Continual pain in lower back, hips or pelvis
- Increased voiding urgency
- Inability to urinate
- Trouble having or keeping an erection (erectile dysfunction)
- Weakness or numbness in the legs or feet

ABOUT THE AUTHOR

Michael J. Dattoli, MD

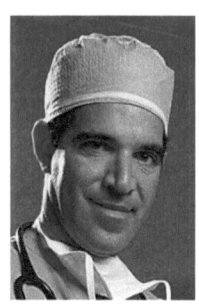

Michael J. Dattoli, MD, is a board-certified radiation oncologist with well over two decades of brachytherapy experience and has performed thousands of prostate implant procedures. He is considered the foremost pioneer in the field, optimizing brachytherapy designs to maximize tumor eradication and minimize symptoms. He has also been the leading trailblazer in the development of Dynamic Adaptive Radiotherapy (DART), utilizing all of the state-of-the-art modalities associated with 4-Dimensional Image-Guided Intensity Modulated Radiotherapy (3D-IMRT). Dr. Dattoli has successfully applied the same technologies to other forms of cancer, including breast, head and neck, GI, GYN, sarcomas and lung malignancies. He is a noted author and speaker in this complex field of medicine.

Dr. Dattoli attended the University of California at Berkeley and was the Valedictorian of his class at Vassar College; he earned his medical degree at Mount Sinai School of Medicine, Radiation Oncology at New York University Medical Center, then distinguished himself at Memorial Sloan-Kettering Cancer Center and New York Hospital-Cornell University Medical Center, as the Special Fellow in Brachytherapy. He was appointed Associate Professor in Brachytherapy and Radiation Oncology at Memorial Sloan- Kettering Cancer Center in New York and at New York Hospital-Cornell University Medical Center prior to relocating to Florida. Dr. Dattoli also serves on multiple journal editorial review boards. Government appointments include "The Prostate Cancer Task Force" in Florida and consultant to the "Washington Oncology Roundtable Advisory Committee". He was selected by the International Association of Oncologists as a Leading Physician of the World and top Brachytherapist.

THE DATTOLI CANCER FOUNDATION MISSION

The Dattoli Cancer Foundation, sponsor of the Prostate Cancer Resource Network, is a 501(c)(3), tax-exempt charitable organization, whose mission is

- to raise awareness of the wide-spread incidence of Prostate Cancer and the need for early and annual screenings;

- to provide information and support to men newly diagnosed with Prostate Cancer as well as to those with recurrent Prostate Cancer, and

- to foster research into better diagnostic tools and treatment options for Prostate Cancer.

Gifts to the Dattoli Foundation make possible publications like this one, and are welcomed anytime. A copy of the official registration and financial information may be obtained from the Division of Consumer Services by calling toll-free (800-435-7352) within the state. Registration does not imply endorsement, approval or recommendations by the state.

Dattoli Cancer Foundation
2803 Fruitville Road
Sarasota, FL 34237
941/365-5599
800/915-1001
fax: 941/330-2317
www.dattolifoundation.org

ORDER MORE BOOKLETS IN THE SERIES

This *Prostate Cancer Essentials for Survival* booklet was published by the Datolli Cancer Foundation. For a complete list of booklets in the series and ordering information, please visit the Dattoli Cancer Center Book Shelf at dattoli.com/book-shelf. Current titles include::

- ✔ Conquering Prostate Cancer with DART and Brachytherapy
- ✔ Dynamic Adaptive Radiation Therapy for Prostate Cancer
- ✔ The Facts: Comparing Prosate Cancer Treatment Options
- ✔ Interpreting Your PSA Results and Related Prostate Cancer Lab Tests
- ✔ Coping with Prostate Cancer Recurrence: Advanced Diagnostics and Treatment Options
- ✔ Image-Guided Prostate Biopsy: When, Why and What to Expect
- ✔ Dosimetry and Prostate Cancer Radiotherapy
- ✔ Advanced Imaging for Prostate Cancer: A Primer on 3D Color-Flow Power Doppler Ultrasound, Multiparametric MRI and CT Fusion Techniques
- ✔ Radiation Safety and Prostate Cancer: Need You Be Concerned?
- ✔ Hormonal Therapy for Prostate Cancer: The Benefits and Risks
- ✔ Lymph Node Positive Prostate Cancer: Advanced Diagnostics and Treatment
- ✔ The Dattoli Blue Ribbon Prostate Cancer Solution: How to Survive and Thrive Without Surgery

www.ingramcontent.com/pod-product-compliance
Lightning Source LLC
Chambersburg PA
CBHW040229220526
45473CB00001B/180